Bre's book is an ide _____)lend of ideas whose time _____ that every time I used cannabis, (always with conscious intention) I always found myself noticing signals and sensations from my body about which parts most "wanted or needed" to be stretched and tuned into. I often wondered if somehow the plant intelligence was communicating with my body intelligence. This magical book brought light to this and a lot more for me.

Brian D. Ridgway, author of *Break Your Self Health Addiction*

Breathe: Your Guide to Cannabis, Yoga, and Spirituality, is a valuable offering that will benefit people who want to awaken their healing and embody their soul. As a Radical Mindfulness expert, I've witnessed the liberation of people from childhood trauma when plant medicine is used. Bre Wolfe shares how this guide can connect you to your core connection. I highly recommend you take her advice.

Daniel Gutierrez, Internationally acclaimed Radical Mindfulness Expert, author of *Radical Mindfulness*

Breathe is a book to educate readers on the sacred use of Cannabis as a tool for awakening, healing, self-love that details the spiritual history of this plant and how when combined with intention and yoga can be a tool for the evolution of humanity.

Brigitte Mars, *author of The Country Almanac of Home Remedies*

Bre Wolfe has created a deeply engaging and illuminative book for those interested in the fast growing field of the healing and transformative aspects of cannabis. Weaving together her expansive personal story with research into the realm of science, the history of cannabis use in ancient cultures, the power and potential of the sacred feminine, and of course the integration of plant medicine with yoga and other meditative modalities, she offers readers new insights into the healing power of cannabis. I was particularly inspired by her insights and experiences into the use of cannabis to bring consciousness into the tissues and cells of the physical body, as well as the emotional and spiritual realms. As someone who has worked in the field of energy healing for many years, I highly recommend this book as a means to go deeper into the fascinating and time-honored use of this powerful sacred medicine.

Sharron Rose, President, Sacred Mysteries Productions, filmmaker, composer, teacher, author of *The Path of the Priestess*, director/producer, Quantum Qi

Bre Wolfe has created a narrative that seamlessly weaves personal storytelling with advanced therapeutic and yogic practices using *Cannabis sativa*. I highly recommend her book to anyone looking for a deeper relationship with this magical plant. It is deeply meaningful to see cannabis honored in this way.

Daniel McQueen, Author of *Psychedelic Cannabis: Breaking the Gate*

In *Breathe: Your Guide to Cannabis, Yoga and Spirituality,* Bre Wolfe provides a guide for being truly alive. Her focus on a practice of breathing, relaxing and movement allow those who work and play with her and her method for awakening to be more aware and to live with mindfulness and intention. Bre reminds the reader of the need to *feel* themselves (not just *think* themselves) and to respect their own voices and lovingly speak their truth. All of this...and more...is a foundation for knowing our creative essence and using our creative voice. I am thoroughly impressed with her authenticity, timeless compassion and creative engagement with what she believes. She lives and writes convincingly about her discoveries and her world. *Breathe* is an insightful and worthwhile read. Enjoy!!

Elsie Ritzenhein, Mentor and Best Selling Author of *Awakening Your Creative Voice*

Run, don't walk, to the nearest computer keyboard and order this book – but only if you want to deepen, accelerate and enliven your journey of inner healing and spiritual growth. Rarely have I read a book that integrates a compelling personal story with tangible experience with clear practical guidance with an impassioned vision of the possible – all for the benefit of those who've begun walking the pathway of feeling, realizing and living the essence of their being.

Ms. Wolfe captures our attention with a personal story of her life-changing exposure to plant medicine, which she calls Santa Maria, and she doesn't let go for the rest of the book. In chapter after chapter she clearly, even beautifully, explains the nature of, research behind, applications of, and tangible effects of plant medicine, especially when it is mindfully and judiciously combined with regular, gentle yoga practice. Together the two practices deepen awareness enormously for participants, both in the moment and then – significantly and decisively – over time as manifested in her own life. Her writing leaves us with no doubt about how the remarkable energy of the two practices elevate consciousness about the self, our connection to all things, and what we can tangibly do to live with greater cognizance and compassion with others and the planet.

Finally, this isn't a book for those who want to imbibe in plant medicine casually and with no deeper intent to grow spiritually. Nor is it for those who know little or nothing about yoga, the language of its techniques and applications, or its historical and spiritual traditions. She clearly explains the latter but assumes a familiarity of the rest that only yoga students are likely to understand and appreciate.

Dr. William Spady, bestselling author of *Outcome-Based Education's Empowering Essence*

BREATHE

Your Guide to Cannabis, Yoga, and Spirituality

Bre Wolfe

BREATHE

Your Guide to Cannabis, Yoga and Spirituality

by Bre Wolfe

Published by Mason Works Press, Boulder, Colorado.
No part of this book may be used or reproduced in any manner
whatsoever without written permission except in the case of
brief quotations embodied in critical articles and reviews.

For information, please contact Kathy Mason, Publisher,
at kathy@masonworksmarketing.com,
or write to Mason Works Press,
6525 Gunpark Dr. #370-426,
Boulder, CO 80301.

Disclaimer: While the publisher and author have used their best
efforts in preparing this book, they make no representations
or warranties with respect to its accuracy or completeness. In
addition, this book contains no legal or medical advice; please
consult a licensed professional if appropriate.

Cover and Interior Design by Kathy Mason and Maryann Sperry

ISBN-13: 978-0-9983209-4-6/ ISBN-10: 0-9983209-4-3

First Edition

Library of Congress Control Number: 2020923001
Published in the United States of America
Printed in the United States of America

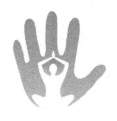

For Brent

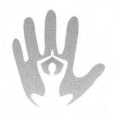

ACKNOWLEDGMENTS

This book would not have been born were it not for the encouragement of my husband Brent. Thank you Brent for everything you've done for me big and small!

And thank you Mary Sojourner for your editing. Your attention to word crafting, detail and flow infused life-giving prana into every page. Thank you Kathy and the team at Mason Works Marketing! It was pure joy working with you!

I want to also thank you, Mommy Dearest, for your unconditional love my entire life. And Dad, for being my biggest teacher. Thank you to my amazing children! All six of you, Moorea, Whitney, Clayton, Cody (and Lexy) Brendan and Keegan. You continue to inspire me by how you listen and follow your heart and your truth. Thank you to my inspiring friends. Your frequency lifts me to ever increasing heights! And to my siblings, Thank you Tanya, Bert, and LaNae. I know you are always there even if we don't always see each other. Also I offer my deep humble gratitude to Bhagavan Krishna, Mahavatar Babaji, Lahiri Mahasaya, Swami Sri Yukteswar

Paramahansa Yogananda, Jesus Christ, Neem Karoli Baba and Mother Teresa.

Lastly, this acknowledgment would not be complete without recognizing my 40,000 brothers and sisters who are currently incarcerated in the United States for marijuana offenses, even as the overall legal cannabis industry is booming.

We are the ones we've been waiting for.

The time is now.

Go outside.

Do it now.

Take this book with you—if you must,

but more importantly,

GET OUTSIDE.

Stop everything else.

Breathe

and

Listen

Outdoors.

The real me wears white all the time. I call everyone brother and sister. I am a steward of the earth. I am light inside a vehicle we call a body. I am calling to you! I recognize you. I see your light. Meet me outside!

TABLE OF CONTENTS

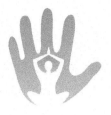

FOREWORD

By Stephen Gray

An image I've had in mind for some time about the current planetary situation—more appropriately labeled a predicament or even a crisis—is that of a vortex. Imagine a boat moving slowly downstream in a river toward a powerful whirlpool. When the boat first gets pulled into the outer edges of the spiral, it circles slowly. With each revolution, the circumference becomes smaller, the pull stronger, and the movement faster.

Humanity is well into the pull of that vortex at this point. In my view, shared by a number of visionaries and mystics I know, there is now nothing stopping our inevitable trajectory toward finally being pulled down into the vortex.

But what does that actually mean in the real world for humanity?

It means that the flatland, business-as-usual days may be pretty much over on this planet. The near- and mid-term future is almost certain to be very challenging. A radical and widespread consciousness transformation is essential, especially for the benefit of the generations to come.

And what does *that* mean, you might ask? To begin with, it implies the inescapable fact that a great majority of humanity has for a long time been disconnected from our natural, unconditional relationship to ourselves, to nature, and to the divine eternal creation altogether.

An essential aspect of that transformation is that we have to re-discover our interwoven, interdependent relationship with plants and in particular with plant medicines. Plants comprise a vast and extensive natural pharmacy. They have been at the center of humanity's survival forever. They are intelligent and we are embedded in their world.

Lo and behold, there just happens to be a plant that is arguably humanity's most intimate ancient friend and ally. The lineage from which this plant comes is estimated to be somewhere between 30 and 90 million years old. It has certainly been with us since the dawn of civilization and has since generously provided us with everything from building materials, to paper, fabric, rope, a base for paints and cosmetics, food, medicine, and, most relevant to the issues addressed in Bre Wolfe's new book, as a spiritual ally.

This book, *Breathe: Your Guide to Cannabis, Yoga, and Spirituality*, is a valuable offering that will benefit any sincere person wanting to work with cannabis—and by association, other psychedelics—as an important component of an ongoing spiritual practice. Bre's own journey of healing and awakening with the assistance of cannabis amply demonstrates the plant's still poorly understood yet remarkable potential, particularly when used skillfully with clear intention and not as an easy escape from the sometimes rugged challenges of being human.

The word "Guide" in the subtitle is an appropriate descriptor for the book. It's an interwoven blend of the personal and the instructional. Bre uses her own experience as the crucible while offering user-friendly information that ranges from an educational tour through some of the historical uses of cannabis for spiritual awakening; to its beneficial partnership with yoga and meditation (including easily applied specific suggestions for practice); to a call to action that takes us beyond our own concerns to compassionate engagement at this crucial juncture in the human story.

As you'll see while reading the book, an absolutely central aspect of this necessary consciousness transformation is the recognition that, with the kind assistance of plant allies like cannabis, we are our own healers. I believe we are far more powerful in this way than almost all of us have known. Bre makes this clear repeatedly with encouraging comments like, "...always listen to you, to your heart and body! Not just in a yoga class, but as you go through your day."

There's a Buddhist principle that the bodhisattva—the compassionate "student teacher" journeying on the path of awakening and helping others along the way—never goes beyond what he or she knows. In that regard I was impressed with Bre's respectful and humble attitude toward the reader. As she says in the book, "I can only share what I practice— what I truly know." Then she invites the reader to take what resonates and leave the rest.

I would trust the advice and guidance of someone who makes statements like those. In the case of *Breathe: Your Guide to Cannabis, Yoga, and Spirituality,* I believe you *can* trust the guidance and make beneficial use of it on your life journey. The great wisdom masters remind us that we're all capable of seeing through illusion and suffering, and then waking up to our true nature as joyful, loving, intelligent sparks of the divine. All the beings of our beloved and beleaguered planet need us to make that journey, now more than ever.

May the path clarify confusion and may confusion dawn as wisdom. —*Buddhist prayer*

—Stephen Gray, Author of *Cannabis and Spirituality: An Explorer's Guide to an Ancient Plant Spirit Ally.*

Stephen Gray is an author/editor, educator, workshop and ceremony leader, conference organizer, and podcast/ YouTube channel host (StephenGray Vision.) Stephen is the author of Returning to Sacred World: A Spiritual Toolkit for the Emerging Reality, and editor/contributor to Cannabis and Spirituality: An Explorer's Guide to an Ancient Plant Spirit Ally.

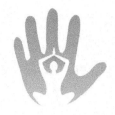

PREFACE

By Joan Bello

M ost books don't have a palpable vibration. This one does.

Bre Wolfe has written the seminal book on the complementary affinity between the practice of yoga and Cannabis as a Spiritual ally. All seekers forward in time will reference her work when studying this ageless, yet hidden, spiritual tradition. Wolfe comes to us with a pedigree of life experience, study, and most importantly from her open heart. It is timely that she makes her appearance at this moment when so many are primed to turn their attention from the trivial to the core values that define our potential.

She is a welcomed channel to help us through these darkest times. As a writer, Wolfe has a rare honesty. You can feel her intent to forge a soul-felt melding with the reader. You know who she is and why she is sharing the rhythm that flows seamlessly across every moment.

In *Breathe: Your Guide to Cannabis, Yoga and Spirituality*, Wolfe has delivered passage to an enchanted pause that cannot ever be forgotten. At the outset, she offers a logical preamble to what is coming, even suggesting which topic might most interest the reader, that one might even skip a section to move forward faster.

But there is no rush. Within the first few pages, Wolfe has set a gentle exhilarating anticipation to follow her lead. She is confident but humble, her tone is accepting, no ego seeps into her message. Rather than instruction, it feels like a sharing in wonder is taking place. The reader is mesmerized by her ability to cut to the chase while maintaining an imperceptible ease of concentration. Her words are deliberate but tender, breathed into the reader's consciousness quite imperceptibly.

No doubt this author is gifted with the art of communicating. She knows exactly how to sequence her topics and answers your questions as though she is reading your mind. As a backdrop to explaining how yoga and marijuana enhance our being, a mystical tempo carries us along. Wolfe is a serious student of Eastern philosophy, clearly an adept at teaching yoga asana, a Devotee of Santa Maria, and a talented, even poetic, writer. Her book inspires and comforts us, while urging us to re-learn what yoga signifies and where marijuana takes us—the ancient marriage.

Breathe: Your Guide to Cannabis, Yoga and Spirituality is tiny compared to the vast tomes of every age. Perhaps because nothing extraneous enters this book, there is room for so much valuable stuff. Makes me realize that there are too many words that fill so many books yet say so little. There is no doubt that Wolfe has been careful to offer only what is necessary. There are no fillers—nothing to distract from the reader's attention. Although she speaks from humility, yet her demeanor is authentic, empowered and calm. Since I had been asked to offer my opinion of this *work,* naturally I paid close attention. Once finished, I sat at my desk to describe what had turned out to be a quite unexpected honor.

I could clearly hear Wolfe's steady voice. She displays a pureness that belies her wealth of knowledge and experience. But when had we spoken? I searched my memory and finally realized that we never had. All personal communication was through the sterility of e-mail. But I heard her. I recognized her. But only from the book! I remembered a brief section toward the end concerning empaths; it stood out because I was unsure why it was there. In hindsight, considering the otherworldly impact her words had on me, I know now that we met on a higher plane.

Chapters build on each other in understanding, so that the whole is greater than the sum of its additions. More is gained than was given. As I said, this is a small book—a quick read, especially if you are as infatuated as I was. Nevertheless, time goes by delightfully slowly, the descriptions of yoga practice enhanced with Cannabis lure the reader into a tranquil, yet energized state. The emotions that she describes in the arms of Cannabis Sativa are authentic, as all of us who love marijuana will immediately perceive. "Blending cannabis with yoga, made me feel as though I was coming home... what flows through me is a synthesis of kundalini, pranayama, asana, and affirmations.... Cannabis smooths the flow.... unlike any yoga .... probably how yoga was practiced.... thousands of years ago." (Chapter Three Teaching Sacred) The veneration of Cannabis has an ancient lineage, uncommon knowledge in modern times.

Obviously, Wolfe was inspired to retrace that history, since her book is by no means just descriptive of her joyous discovery of the effects of our sacred plant. The reader is treated to a brief but fulsome explanation of the most salient points that she ferreted out from the wisdom of the sages: "I explored the history of the pairing of cannabis and yoga...found out that when combined, cannabis, yoga and spirituality is not new.... It's been used as an ally to help humankind ponder deeply religious and philosophical subjects." (Chapter Two History of Cannabis, Yoga and Spirituality) She cites examples from Buddhism, Hinduism, Taoism, along with present day Rastafarians, and more. Her precise explanation of *The Vedas* displays her scholarly mastery.

It seems that no stone has been left unturned when it comes to the stated topic of Wolfe's book. It is all here. In addition, she gives us the usual snapshot of her outer world, shares with us psychological traumas and such, simultaneously, her melodic voice bears witness to her reactions to herself. We learn how the consciousness, imparted by her yogic practices of asana, intentionality, attentional breathing, and meditation had served her/ saved her for decades as she navigated through her personal chaos. She describes in vivid detail the transformative enhancement that took place with the addition of cannabis to her practice. Her meditations became effortless, her practice of yoga asana was infused with more strength of awareness, more gratitude, more ease. Describing the delayed *high* will resonate with every marijuana devotee: "Something is happening.... I can go deeper into this body.... feel more. Passing through to another place feels like swimming through a waterfall.... I pop up on the other side. I'm not aware of there being sides. There is just being."

She is a wonderfully adept yoga teacher. In Chapter five, "How You Might Experience a Sacred Plant Medicine Class," the reader is led through a full session. Just by reading her words, we see the class, we hear the bells, we are empowered and relaxed. As a personal note, I want to report that I have taken many a yoga class, many guided by a trained instructor's voice, most of which in secret companionship with cannabis. None have resonated in my being with such delight as the one led by Bre Wolfe. "When cannabis and intentions are combined, the results of meditation are amplified. Santa Maria infuses your intention with greater power."

In no period in modern history has the turning to spiritual truths been more pronounced, harkened to more people, and with more urgency than now. In this tumultuous reality, there is the irresistible yearning for help. If each of us yokes our soul in harmony, lives and breathes deeply, freely, joyfully in everlasting gratitude for the blessing of Santa Maria in homage to the sages who left us their treasure of yoga, we will be heeding the purpose, mission, and tenets of Wolfe's book. We can follow her steady voice that breathes into us from her heart.

This book is inspired by the spirit of our magical Plant Medicine. The reader feels the invisible vibrancy guiding the author. Her words are deliberate but gentle, synced with the reader's consciousness quite imperceptibly. No doubt she has been gifted with the art of communicating. There is a magical flow to her writing, a felt rhythm that carries us beyond ourselves.

To say that *Cannabis Sativa* changed Bre Wolfe is correct. She became herself. It is my pleasure to know her. Marijuana changed my life also. I have known many on this same irresistible road. Wolfe offers us a way of learning to be on the path to ourselves. She is taking the journey with the reader and when you close this book, you realize she is taking the journey for the reader, as well. Sisters and Brothers who are what this book is all about, this is a moment to rejoice. We have been blessed with an eloquent Soul-Sister.

Joan Bello, author of *The Benefits of Marijuana: Physical, Psychological & Spiritual,* is incredibly courageous and brilliant in her presentation of marijuana as the SUPREME HOLISTIC MEDICINE. Her hypothesis, that marijuana balances the Autonomic Nervous System—which then sets the stage for health beyond the ordinary—is in keeping with the tenets of Yoga Science. Her expertise was garnered through vigorous academic training in a specialized Master of Science Program accessible to only a few hand-chosen students. She is fulfilling her mandate of bringing the Eastern wisdom to the West in this revolutionary handling of the abiding connection between esoteric discipline and the state of consciousness fostered with marijuana.

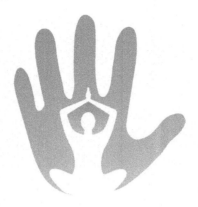

PART 1

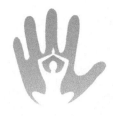

PROLOGUE

"When will you begin that long journey into yourself?" —Rumi

My husband, Brent, and I have been invited to dinner with our new friends, Lela and Drew, in a luxurious ski-chalet home in Telluride, Colorado. Although it's only six in the evening, it's dark and freezing outside, but I'm warm by a crackling fire. Brent and our host and hostess are in the kitchen. I treasure these few moments of solitude, moments during which I am free to do nothing.

There are appetizers on the low table in front of me: aged cheeses, kalamata olives, whole grain crackers and little bowls of chocolates and candies. There is a glass of a deep red wine. A crystal bowl directly in front of me holds a rainbow of gum drops—red, green, yellow. I reach for a couple. I'm about to pop them in my mouth when Lela looks out of the kitchen.

"Take just one, Bre. They're loaded."

Loaded? These must be marijuana gum drops. It is January 2014, and Colorado has just legalized cannabis for recreational use. I'm curious and wary. Should I have one? What if I feel too much? What if I see too much, what if I see things I don't like in the other people—in myself. That's what happened years ago when I got high for the first time in high school. I had told myself I would never try pot again.

That night I woke to a voice that seemed real. "Bre, do not do this again. Now is not the time for you. This could cause irreparable damage to your brain. There will come a time when this medicine will be helpful for you." The voice was more real than a dream. All of that was so long ago and I had completely forgotten about it until this moment.

Lela sits down across from me. "I am going to try *one*," I say, "but if I act weird or get quiet, please don't take it personally. It won't be about you."

She laughs gently and says, "Drew and I do this all the time—sometimes by ourselves, sometimes with other people. Start with just half the gummy and see how you feel. I'll be right here with you."

"I'm not sure," I say. "The last time I tried pot in high school, I got super paranoid." I shake my head back and forth. "It was terrible."

The men join us on the overstuffed leather couches. Both of them grab a gummy and casually pop it into their mouth. My husband says, "Are you going to try one?"

"I think so."

Lela smiles. "It's going to be fine. But that salmon isn't going to be if I don't get it out of the oven."

I wonder if she is high. All I've seen her do is sip a little wine. I'd feel safer with her if I knew she hadn't partaken. Lela goes into the kitchen. My husband and Drew resume their conversation.

I take a deep breath. The men aren't paying attention. I look at the gummies. Red, green, yellow. *I always liked green.* I hold the gummy between my fingers for a second and then I bite it in half.

Lela calls Drew into the kitchen. A few minutes later, they emerge with a gorgeous salad, and the huge salmon on a platter. Brent and I join them at the dining room table. The meal is elegant and relaxed. Nothing seems different to me. We close the evening with home-churned mango ice cream and tiny cups of espresso.

I don't feel any different than I usually do. We say our goodbyes. Brent and I walk back home through the crisp mountain air. It's not until he and I are getting ready for bed that I notice that my routine of brushing my teeth and taking off my make-up has been replaced by the need to meditate. Something is happening. I usually meditate in the morning.

I climb the stairs to the loft, sit cross-legged, straighten my spine, and feel everything slow down. I watch my breath move steadily in and out like slow waves. I go deeper. Into stillness.

I don't need to concentrate on breathing at all. Without knowing how I am doing it, I make my inhales and exhales so long and so light, that I'm barely aware I'm breathing.

I am free. I am expansive. I am floating. I am light. *I am being breathed.* I look upward behind my closed lids and focus on the center between my eyebrows. There is an intention. I want to experience oneness. I pass through.

Passing through to another place feels like swimming through a waterfall. I plunge through a cascade of electric-gleaming white energy and pop up on the other side. I'm actually not aware of there being sides. There is just being.

I see. I feel. Cool, dark, rich, moist air, growth, ferns, water, possibility. I am in a deeply serene healing place. My cells open and are hydrated. The air is easy to breathe. It's saturated with nutrients that soothe my lungs and skin. I know that breath brought me here.

Although my physical eyes are closed, I "see" baby ferns, greenery and newly formed rocks that look like lava. I am in a rainforest. I am in the physical representation of the energy of peace, ease, hope, and possibility. In an instant I know why rainforests need protection. They are nurseries carefully nurturing thousands of delicate life forms. A hush permeates this delicate nursery and I promise to do all I can to protect it.

I am being nurtured and restored as well. I linger here, I breathe here. For what seems an endless time...I don't know how long I am in that blessed place. Eventually, the feeling of needles in my legs remind me that I am meditating in a loft in the Colorado mountains. Instantly, I leave the rainforest and see me from above, sitting cross-legged on the floor in the loft. I see the back of my head and hair. I'm wearing my favorite cream-colored robe.

There's a whoosh—and I'm back in my body. It feels as though I am wearing a heavy, densely padded snowsuit.

Every part of me is enveloped in stifling layers. I realize for the first time in my life that I-am-feeling-my-body-as-it-really-is. And I know, with calm certainty, that this body? The body I have lived with my whole life? It is not me.

I look at me from inside, just as I would look at the inside of a car I was considering for purchase. I see concaved lungs, an overworked tired heart, polluted rivers of blood in my veins and I see dark decay around my digestive organs. Energetically, I feel like I am sitting in an armored tank.

I concentrate fiercely and take a breath, a slow deep inhale and hold it until my lungs are ready to burst. I forcefully expel the breath—and feel the remarkable sensation of abundant space in my body. I am exhaling what I don't need. I can go deeper into this body of mine so I can feel more. I settle in farther.

There is no I. There is only She who I am exploring. I straighten her body and feel her spine. I notice she needs to tuck in her tailbone and roll her shoulders back so her spine can be as straight as possible. I realize this creates an antenna of sorts and makes her a better receiver to subtle energies.

I raise her arms sideways, parallel to her shoulders, and extend them left and right equally. I am free to know that one can reach past one's fingertips.

I begin to understand. We reach past our fingertips so we can feel the energy-flow all the way past the tips of our fingers. It is simple. That way, we give circulation and life force to every square inch of this vehicle, which I've named my body.

BREATHE

A mountain of truth rises. I am a being of light, wearing a bodysuit so that I can inhabit this biosphere. This body is evolutionarily designed to carry me about as I do my work. BUT THE BODY IS NOT WHO I AM.

My solitary cannabis and meditation/yoga routine becomes my weekly touchstone to myself. I feel I am being roused from a coma. I am waking up. It is as though the morning sun rises, slowly unthawing a carefully constructed, tightly packed personality. As my core softens on the inside, I feel lighter and brighter on the outside. Even though I am only partaking in cannabis once a week, I am feeling changes every day. Little things aren't bothering me. I'm not reacting, I'm observing. I'm far less impatient. I am more relaxed all over.

Cannabis and yoga are teaching me that the tension in my body has been covering my lightness. I can loosen the constriction of my suffocating bodysuit by releasing anything that creates tension in my thoughts. My tense thoughts create the constriction in my body.

I see what it is like to not only feel my body, but to also feel my spirit again. To feel me again. Some gentle part of me has come back and she's staying for longer periods of time.

With this softening comes awareness. One of the earliest things I feel is that I'm suffocating. I haven't breathed properly in so long, that literally I am dying. I close my eyes and see the inside of my body. Cells have been denied adequate amounts of oxygen for so long. They are shriveled and contracted; many are black, like tiny dried-out raisins.

They are floating around in my body, in the murky, swampy rivers of my blood. I have been poisoning myself.

So, each day, whenever I need to, I take breaths! I breathe in deep, slow inhales through the nose. I fill my lungs full and hold the blessed air until I'm prompted by my body to let it go. I push the air out with force and know I am expelling toxicity. I do this over and over until my lungs feel like they have an adequate supply of clean, life-giving oxygen. I understand that breathing like this is necessary to keep the blood rivers in my body flowing.

While I'm breathing, my body naturally moves into certain yoga poses to help me expel stiffness in my joints or stagnation in my organs. I fold forward in uttanasana and dangle for a long time there. I feel it restoring and expanding my lungs. Or, I sit in baddha konasana, bringing needed circulation to my stomach, ovaries, bladder, and kidneys. I continue breathing in different ways and in different patterns throughout my practice. I learn more about how this practice, my practice, keeps everything moving; how it releases toxicities in my body and influences from my past.

I move to the point where I feel my body almost all the time. I see how negative thinking, bad attitudes, and fear affect it. I feel thoughts that cause me to contract. I see how they add darkness and heaviness in me and my body bit by bit. I realize when my breathing slows, my thoughts in accordance slow. When my thoughts speed up, my breath accelerates and becomes shallow. I want to stay in peace, so I do everything I can to breathe mindfully and go slow. I am healing my broken spirit and my wounded body.

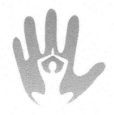

USER'S MAP

"The spiritual journey is individual, highly personal. It can't be organized or regulated. It isn't true that everyone should follow one path. Listen to your own truth." —*Ram Dass*

N amaste,

I imagine that if you have found this book, opened it, and read as far as this map, you are looking for something in your life that seems to be missing. I imagine that you are either starting out on finding a path to what you don't as yet know you need; or you have explored many practices and still feel an emptiness, a longing, an ache for knowledge, and an experience you have lost.

Welcome.

To help you navigate this book's sources of knowledge, personal experience, scientific fact, imaginings, and hope,

I invite you to leaf through this book and pay attention to when you feel curious; when a word or words touch you. Read for a while. Then pause, let that soak in. Begin to feel the message. Then let yourself go farther. This guide can help you find what you may be looking for.

For instance, if you want to learn more about the gifts of a yoga and cannabis practice, go to Chapter four. If you need to understand the psychology and brain chemistry of cannabis use, go to Chapter Ten. If you want to meet the writer, go to the Prologue and Chapter One. Are you curious about a short multi-cultural history of the use of cannabis as a sacrament and meditation tool? Chapter Two opens that window.

Each chapter leads to the next; each piece of knowledge opens doors to more understanding. And, if you want to learn how I evolved the practice of melding yoga and intelligent, mindful cannabis use, begin with Chapter Three.

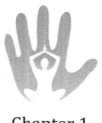

Chapter 1

MY LIFE STORY-
UP TILL THIS MOMENT

"We shall not cease from exploration and the end of all our exploring will be to arrive where we started and know the place for the first time."—T.S. Elliot

W hen I was set out on my journey, I had no idea that the peace, security, and love I had experienced in my early childhood would ever be shattered. As a little girl, I had felt deep love and gratitude for everyone and everything, especially nature. I had no idea that there would come a time where I'd experience myself with utter disgust and punish myself for everything and anything I could possibly blame on me. I had no idea I would reach a place so low I'd want to discard myself.

And, I didn't know that my self-loathing would bring me to an even deeper realization of love and supreme connection with all things. I had no idea or sense that it would take me losing everything I ever dreamed I'd wanted—in order to find that which was always there inside me, waiting to be acknowledged.

Only after I destroyed my life and lost that which I held most dear—my family, my cherished children, my salt-of-the-earth husband, my career, all the things I believed that I had spent my lifetime creating—was I finally forced to look at the one person I had learned to hate. And, she was the person I saw when I could bear to look in a mirror.

I didn't know who she was. I didn't know why I hated her. I had spent my life trying to be "everything" I thought "everyone" expected me to be. I became the best television newscaster I could be, the best wife, the best mother, the best, most perfect friend and daughter. I gave away *who I* was. And, I had no idea how to find that girl/woman I had lost.

I know now that I was not alone in that form of a soul give-away.

I grew up in Nome, Alaska on the Bering Sea, part of a Caucasian minority in an Inupiat Eskimo village of about two thousand people. I was blessed to spend long summers in the midnight sun, camping and fishing and jumping from rock to rock on the seawall that protected the town from the ocean. We kids spent winters building forts and jumping off roof tops into huge snowdrifts that were sometimes higher than the homes themselves. My older sister Tanya would lead the way and my twin brother Bert and I would follow. We would take turns climbing and jumping over and over. Little LaNae, my baby sister, loved watching us. She and I would make snow angels in the fresh powder after every blizzard.

Or, we would ice skate on ponds of crystalline-clear ice. When we got tired from skating, we would lie face down on the ice. Once our eyes got accustomed to the dark water beneath, we could see fish frozen in place directly below us. They were still alive but held in place until the spring thaw. That seemed miraculous, but I had learned that Mother Earth takes care of us and how connected we all are to her and all of life. I see now how that early childhood in nature was the precious gift of a foundation that kept me rooted.

Our family didn't belong to a church. My mother encouraged my brother and sisters and me to visit different ones so we could pick the one that resonated most with us. Despite the fact that our town was small, when it came to churches, we had Catholic, Methodist, Protestant, Lutheran, Pentecostal, Baptist and even Baha'i Faith. I went to all of them. I found it didn't really matter what the exact teaching was. I felt God in each of them, But I felt *Her* the most when I was outside.

The only major ongoing difficulty I experienced as a child was with my father. As hard as I tried, I never could please him. No one could. He was a bush pilot and under a lot of pressure from flying in dangerous weather conditions. When he was home, I felt as though I never knew what was going to set him off and get him upset.

I constantly tried to please him. He was my hero. But he never seemed happy. He never gave any of us a compliment or approved of anything. His criticism made me try harder to be more perfect. With a child's logic I figured if I tried harder to please him, he would finally be happy. I kept thinking, "If I am perfect, then he will love me—he will love us."

Then, around the time I was twelve, my father crashed his plane during take-off. His plane had lifted off the ground and was climbing when the engine cut out. He tried to bank it, but the plane cartwheeled and plummeted like an arrow to the ground. Once it hit, the right wing continued to spin, then the fuselage broke apart just behind the baggage compartment. My father survived with just a broken collar bone. His one passenger on that particular flight also survived.

Dad had always been my definition of courage. He was my Father. By surviving the crash, it confirmed for me that he was indeed the superman I always secretly believed he was. I vowed harder to make him happy.

Shortly after the crash, my parents decided to move our family to Phoenix, Arizona. I was now thirteen—and Arizona seemed as far away to me as any place I could imagine. I had only seen pictures of Arizona deserts with cactus and western movies with shootouts and horses. I wondered if living there meant we would have to ride horses to school. I was excited at the prospect of exploring lands and people outside of the tundra and freezing cold I knew.

We all adjusted to life in the huge city of Phoenix and I thought we were happy—until one day I came home from school and was surprised to find my Dad waiting for me. He was always working and certainly never home in the day.

We went outside by the white picket fence that lined our yard and he said the last thing I wanted to hear.

"Honey. I have been unhappy for a long time and I want to let you know, I am moving out. I wanted to tell you because

I knew you would understand. I met another woman who I've grown to love and I am moving in with her. I'd like you to explain this to your brother and sisters for me."

I was 14 years old.

I nodded my head yes, like a robot, like the good girl I was raised to be. Then my father gave me a fast, hard hug, jumped into the family station wagon, and drove away.

Later that night, I numbly recited what I was told to my brother and sisters. That is when my older sister told me the other reason we had moved from Alaska.

"Bre, you know why we moved here to Phoenix, don't you?" she said.

"What are you talking about?" She wasn't making sense. I was talking about Dad leaving us, here and now, and she was talking about why we left Nome.

She blurted it out. "Dad had been having affairs on Mom."

Bert chimed in, "I saw him kissing Mary once."

"Ya, but that was as a friend," I protested. I had seen him kiss her myself too. "It was like adults that kiss friends."

I felt sick. My stomach hurt. *My parents not only wanted to leave the harsh Alaskan winters, they were trying to give their marriage a fresh start.*

My storybook childhood was over. I felt I had been lied to my whole life and my Dad had cheated not only on Mom, but on me—on us. He had been my brave fighter. He had been my rock. To me he had no faults. Even if I never felt like I was good enough for him.

My Mom and siblings never really talked about my father's affairs again. We never talked about anything. We all just carried on. I rarely ever saw my Dad after that. I continued going to school and got as involved in it as I could. I found out if I stayed busy, I didn't have to feel.

No dad. Numb. Mom started working two jobs to make ends meet. This was change I hadn't asked for. But, one constant remained. Food. I'd come home at night from my job or from being out with friends and rummage through the cupboards and refrigerator. I didn't know exactly what I was looking for. Invariably, I'd settle on something sweet, something sugary.

I'd start with a teeny bite. Then, with that bite, something would take over. I'd tell myself, it's okay to take a second bite. And then I'd say, three bites are fine and that's it. Somewhere after that, I'd lose track.

I'd come to and realize with panic that I'd eaten an entire pie, cake, a bag of cookies. I felt as though I was full of repulsive slime. I had to get rid of it. The only way to get it out of me was to throw it up. I didn't know why I did it. And I didn't know how to stop it. I felt horrifyingly ashamed. And, I had no one to talk to.

A caring teacher must have sensed my pain and confusion, because he gave me a book that altered the course of my life forever. It was *The Relaxation Response* by Dr. Herbert Benson. That tiny yellow book was my introduction to a lifetime of meditation. *The Relaxation Response* is a simple, secular version of Transcendental Meditation ("TM"), presented for people in the Western world. Summer break was just starting and I decided I would experiment with meditating for the summer. I decided to follow the directions in the book and meditate every morning just to see if anything happened. My mantra was the word "One." I had specifically chosen the number "one" because it had no religious ties to it.

I practiced so consistently that within two months, the minute I would sit in silence, I'd instantly drop into deep relaxation. One morning towards the end of summer, I breathed in my mantra. As I silently repeated my mantra, I felt myself getting lighter, weightless. I felt myself vibrating. I saw how *everything* continually vibrated with intelligence. I saw everything was energy and *we are all one*. I had always thought one was just a number.

After that event, I was compelled to find out what I had experienced. I needed to know more about all things being one energy. That occurrence and my curiosity started my lifelong pursuit of learning about and understanding consciousness.

I continued meditating through high school. As I continued my meditation, my bulimia eased. It would rear up now and then—only when I got out of balance. I learned that if I over-committed and went too fast from one activity to the next without pauses to feel myself and rest, my balance would slip.

The next major event that shaped who I am, and what I teach now, was so little that I didn't really notice it until years later. I was seventeen, a senior in high school. I spent the night at a girlfriend's house—specifically so we could try marijuana. We got a joint from her brother and he showed us how to light it and inhale.

The pot hit me right away. I instantly felt suspicious, insecure, and overwhelmed with everything. I wanted to go home and I did. I went up to bed, but I couldn't relax. When I finally managed to fall asleep that night, I was awakened by whispers and low murmurings from a group of people who seemed to be hovering near the foot of my bed, near the corner wall. The sensation was weird, scary, and disconcerting.

I quickly reached for the lamp beside my bed and turned it on. There was no one in my room. I calmed myself, turned off the lamp, lay back down and realized the voices were coming from somewhere deep inside me. It felt like a counsel of people coming out in one collective voice. They were authoritative in a concerned way.

"Bre, Bre, Bre," they implored, "do not do this again. Do not do this anymore right now. This will be detrimental for you if you do this now. *The time is not right.*" I understood somehow that smoking marijuana at that point would cause some kind of harm in my life—possibly to my brain—and that the practice could affect me in adverse ways if I engaged in it at that point in my life.

"How come this seems so real to me, and I have no doubt you are really talking to me, and that this is not my imagination?" I thought.

I was "told" that: "There will be a time when this *is* right for you. It will be a long time from now." I saw a vague picture in my head of me in a distant, indistinct future—nothing like the crystalline silent conversation I was having with the voices. The warning was so strong and real, however, that I wrote the experience in my diary. As time went on, I forgot about it. I had no temptation to try marijuana again for a long, long time. Drugs and alcohol had never been my thing and did not become important in my life.

For the next twenty years I pursued my interests. I worked full time while going to college. I studied Journalism Broadcasting and loved it because I learned new things every day—and broadcast journalism gave me license to talk to people from all walks of life.

While I was in college, I discovered another book that influenced my life, *You Can Heal Your Life*, by Louise Hay. She has written about how specific thoughts and thought patterns create corresponding specific dis-eases in the body. It made brilliant sense to me, so I started testing her theory on myself and family and with my friends and associates.

Anytime someone complained about a sickness or ailment, I'd look up the condition and read the thought pattern associated with that dis-ease. They were always a match.

I looked up my own symptoms and found bulimia defined *metaphysically* as "hopeless terror. A frantic stuffing and purging of self-hatred." Hay helped me realize and understand my self-talk—the way I talked to myself silently in my head. It wasn't pretty.

Her book taught me to instead use affirming, gentle, and loving words when I talked to myself. To challenge my bulimia, I started affirming, "I am loved and nourished and supported by Life itself. It is safe for me to be alive."

Hay's book showed me that our words are powerful—and we constantly create our experiences based on what we think and what we say. I learned from her that we create what we talk about. If I spend my time complaining about what is not working, I will create more of what is not working. I learned from her to constantly look for the gift in every perceived hardship.

I went to my first Hatha Yoga class with my boyfriend when I was in my late 20s. I loved it. It felt like I had come home into my body—with love and with compassion. For the first time, I could sit in my physical body—as it was—and just breathe. Sometimes in certain postures my tears would come out. I didn't know then that our trauma can get stuck and trapped in our tissues. I just knew I felt release...and lighter when I walked out of class.

I understand now that the shifts created by reading and practicing what I was learning and taking part in happened below the radar. They occurred while I was busy living, pursuing my career and pursuing the American dream along with all the material trappings of success.

I married my yoga companion. Two years later I graduated college, turned 30 and became pregnant with our first son, Brendan. I landed a job in a small television market. My infant son and I moved to Helena, Montana, while my husband commuted from Phoenix.

Instantly the pressure was on. I was now a single mother in a new town, working at my new broadcasting career. It was just the baby and me until the weekend came. My husband would fly in on Fridays and Brendan and I would take him back to the airport Monday morning.

The airfare ate up all the money my husband earned. I made just enough to pay for childcare and a small, dark basement apartment. Our little family wore used clothing and followed a strict budget. But we were making it happen.

Within six months I made it to a bigger market in Colorado Springs. They offered me the main anchor position for the five and ten PM newscasts. It was fun and exciting and stimulating and nonstop. My husband and I commuted for five more years.

During that time, there never was any time for sitting and resting. I was running—running on adrenaline. I fueled my excitement and exhaustion by living off mocha lattes and Krispy Kreme donuts. Because they are both high in calories, I'd skimp on other foods. I figured calories were just calories. I didn't think for a moment about what I might have been doing to my body—to my being.

Although I loved my job, my husband and I both agreed that I would not renew my contract when it expired. We had been commuting our entire marriage and wanted to live together full time, like a real family. We planned on moving back to Phoenix when my contract was up. We figured I had enough experience and if I was lucky, I could probably get a news job in Phoenix.

Shortly after moving back there, I was ecstatic to find out I was pregnant with our second child, Keegan. But, along with that pregnancy came postpartum depression. I know now that it was fueled by a complete depletion of nutrients in my body and huge hormonal changes that accompany pregnancy and birth. I ate well when I was pregnant, but the five years of my caffeine and sugar regimen leading up to the pregnancy didn't leave reserves in my nutrient tank.

The baby had to get what he needed to grow and develop, which meant there was not much of anything left over to fuel me. I was low in energy and I was down. This is when all the feelings I had been running from my entire life emerged. I couldn't run from them. I couldn't run from exhaustion and fear. Our beautiful house felt like a cage.

I felt as though I was drowning in bottles, diapers, and monotony. I thought once I got back into broadcasting, I would feel better. But that wasn't the case.

I was hired by the ABC affiliate in Phoenix and although it felt great to be back working stories, I couldn't shake the dark cloud hovering around me. For a false relief, I tangled myself up in an affair. It didn't escape me that my father had done just that very same thing.

I tried to stop the affair but couldn't. My husband and I saw a marriage counselor, who declared I was a love addict and that people generally become love addicts due to a past history of abandonment from their primary caregivers. He said I showed the classic symptoms: a conscious fear of abandonment with an underlying subconscious fear of intimacy.

His diagnosis was spot on. But I was in denial. It was hard for me to reconcile that it was me having these problems, that I was the one creating all this turmoil and pain. I couldn't end the affair. My beloved husband and I divorced. I lost my job in news because I couldn't concentrate. I moved into a condo I could afford in a rougher part of town.

The minute my marriage was over, I was no longer drawn to the other man. I couldn't believe I created this roller coaster, drama-filled nightmare, that it was me doing these things. Many times, I woke in the night in a panic, not able to breathe. I had constant nightmares I was being chased by dead pirates and skeletons. I'd wake up saying the Lord's prayer and I would repeat it over and over.

Despite my panic, I remembered the truth that we can only concentrate on one thought at a time, so I would concentrate on my inhales and exhales. I was able to quiet my panicking scared self by focusing on the act of breathing.

I felt my breath. And I started watching it in my mind's eye as I breathed. I did nothing else but feel and *see* air come in through my nose and then exit out of my mouth. Focusing on that simple action would bring me to the present moment and *was I okay in this present moment? Yes? Okay, then I could inhale again.*

I started to really pay attention to what I was feeling in my body—all the different sensations. I knew I was at the bottom. Nothing mattered except my children and survival. My counselor graciously still wanted to work with me even though I couldn't pay her. She helped me get in touch with my past and all the feelings I had been afraid to feel—including the profound love I had for my children.

I discovered (or it found me!) a book called *The Dark Side of The Light Chasers*, by Debbie Ford. It is based off Carl Jung's shadow work. This brilliant psychoanalyst taught that everyone carries a shadow and the less a person is consciously aware of it, the blacker and denser the shadow can be. Our shadow is made up of the parts of ourselves we deny, our so-called negative traits, like our crankiness or selfishness. Our shadow can also be our denied brilliance and our denied light. Jung believed and taught that humans need to integrate all parts of our self to be whole.

I read everything I could on the subject, and I practiced what I was learning. As I healed my pain and tried to reconcile my actions, I realized that I wanted to help others with their traumas and pain. I felt like if I could help others avoid the misery I created in my own life, then at least the suffering I had caused my husband and children would not be in vain.

Meditation, yoga, and feeling my body became my anchor to the present moment. I started eating lighter foods and embraced a vegetarian diet because it felt better.

The author, Debbie Ford, also offered Professional Life Coaching certification training. I found supplemental jobs working for the airlines and doing voice-overs and commercials, which helped me pay for the training. Combining these part-time jobs allowed me to work around my children's schedules.

I moved slowly and watched and felt my feelings. When I felt panic coming on, I practiced breathing. Bit by bit the brightness I had known as a child returned.

Eight years after my divorce, I met a man who had a similar outlook as mine. We got our yoga teaching cer-tifications together. We married and continued to raise our kids, though most were in college and high school by this time, except for Keegan, the youngest. When he became an exchange student to Switzerland his junior year of high school, we took the opportunity to live in Telluride, Colorado.

In Telluride, we explored vast mountain hiking trails and ski runs and starry nights and wildflowers that blanketed hillsides. We also had unprecedented time to explore profound inner states through the plant medicine (cannabis) and yoga.

When we returned to Arizona a year later, I created the first in-studio yoga and cannabis class in the state. I taught cannabis yoga for a year in Phoenix before the opportunity to move to Maui, Hawaii presented itself.

A lot has happened in a short time. I started by offering my same humble plant medicine yoga classes in Maui at a healing center. As of this writing, my husband and I have lived in Maui for two years. My classes and offerings have grown. I discovered a community of like-minded people here who understand the myriad and profound gifts cannabis offers.

I also joined an international group of pioneering holistic teachers and therapists based out of Boulder, Colorado. They are part of an intentional psychedelic community that promotes safe and intentional psychedelic medicine practices for personal and global healing and transformation. They offer cannabis-assisted psychedelic therapy for trauma resolution, life transitions, and psychedelic integration support. I will tell you more about their life changing offerings at the end of this book.

When I was undergoing training at a weeklong intensive for cannabis assisted therapy, I experienced another profound vision that brought me full circle to the first time I tried marijuana. In this vision I saw myself in my childhood bedroom. I was lying in my bed, the same bed I was lying in when I heard the "voices" speaking to me the first time I tried marijuana. This time, with this vision, I was not frightened. I clearly felt only deep love and concern coming from the indistinct shapes and outlines of forms hovering around me. I "saw" I had reached the time they had told me about those many years before.

"This is the time," they whispered. "You have arrived at the time. This is to be of great benefit for you and for the world."

I "saw" the same indistinct outlines of shapes hovering over me as if I were still lying in my childhood bed. But, this time, I recognized who they were/are. It hit me with clarity and my heart swelled in recognition.

These concerned beings "talking" to me when I had first tried plant medicine were my grandparents and great-grandparents and their great-grandparents. *They are my ancestors.* They are my kin. They have been watching over me my entire life and they watch over me now.

My vision shifted and I saw that I am physically and energetically being carried on their shoulders. The ground I walk on today is made up from their physical bodies. They are the dust in the earth and they make up the earth. And they whisper to me, "Wake. Have courage. Meditate. Listen. Act. And share."

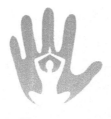

Chapter 2

HISTORY OF CANNABIS, YOGA AND SPIRITUALITY

"Believe nothing, no matter where you read it, or who said it, no matter if I have said it, unless it agrees with your own reason and your own common sense."
—Buddha

When I first experienced the blissfully expansive connection I felt during my cannabis-yoga initiation, I sensed that I had discovered the secrets to the universe. Practicing with cannabis and yoga was far beyond my earlier meditation practices—because it made my spirituality real. It brought the ethereal down into my body where I could feel it. Cannabis intensified my connection with Spirit so I could no longer deny Spirit's existence. Cannabis yoga gave me a key that opened a door into feeling real love for my physical being—and for everything and everyone. I needed to know if anyone else felt this way when they combined plant medicine with a spiritual practice. I knew I needed to research this miracle.

I explored the history of the pairing of cannabis and yoga and I was shocked and surprised. I was shocked because, although I had been doing yoga for more than twenty years, no one in my circles ever talked about practicing the spiritual discipline with cannabis. And I was surprised because, once I put sacred plant, breath, and body together, I intuitively knew they belonged. I found out that when combined, cannabis, yoga, and spirituality is *not* new. In fact, it appears to be as old as humanity's longing for wisdom.

History shows, the cannabis sativa plant has been used by many traditional religious groups as well as shamanic and pagan cultures. It's been used as an ally to help humankind ponder deeply religious and philosophical subjects related to their tribe or society; to achieve a form of enlightenment; to unravel unknown realms and connections of the human mind and subconscious.

Cannabis in Taoism

According to *The Encyclopedia of Cultivated Plants*, cannabis was used as medicine in Asia for at least three thousand years. One of the earliest examples of cannabis use in religion or spirituality can be found in Taoism, the ancient Chinese belief system that dates back to the fourth century BCE. Taoism is based on the philosophy of Lao Tzu and became the official religion of China under the Tang Dynasty, which ruled between 618-907 CE.

Beginning in the fourth century CE, Taoist texts mention using cannabis in censers, which are incense burners. According to the Taoist encyclopedia Wushang Biyao, which means "Supreme Secret Essentials," ancient Taoists experimented regularly with "hallucinogenic smokes." Cannabis reportedly was used to eliminate selfish desires; induce feelings of well-being; and achieve a state of naturalness that corresponded with the core Taoist beliefs. Taoist priests and shamans would combine cannabis with ginseng and use it as a means to communicate with good and evil spirits, as well as to forecast the future. They believed cannabis had the ability to cast one's spirit forward in time. Its use however appears to be limited to priests, shamans, and other holy men. Around 2000 BCE, cannabis spread from Central Asia to India. There are several prominent stories surrounding its widespread acceptance and about the reverence Indians had and still have for cannabis.

Cannabis in Hinduism

One significant story about cannabis use appears in *The Vedas*, another in The Yoga Sutras—both ancient manuscripts are revered in India as authoritative and holy texts that best describe how to live in the physical world without getting caught up in it. Both books are among the oldest known body of information in existence and are the foundational source behind the development of yogic philosophy and Hinduism.

The word "Vedas" translates into the word "knowledge." *The Vedas* are a collection of four books with ancient teachings that are still relevant today. Ancient Vedism is what has shaped modern Hinduism today. *The Vedas* reference the herb as *a source of happiness, a joy-giver, and liberator that was compassionately given to humans to delight the senses and eliminate fear.*

Lord Shiva is one of the principle Gods worshipped in Hinduism. He is considered the lord of cannabis—or bhang, as it's also called in India. Shiva is generally recognized by Hindus and most of India as a lover of the cannabis plant. Often in many of the statues and paintings of Shiva, he holds a bundle of herbs or a pipe.

According to legend, Shiva wandered off into the fields after an angry discourse with his family. Drained from the family conflict and the hot sun, he fell asleep under a leafy plant. When he awoke, he noticed the plant wasn't wilting in the hot sun. His curiosity led him to sample the leaves and he became rejuvenated and refreshed.

Cannabis soon became a preferred part of Shiva's diet. Cannabis was so satisfying to him that he even declared it his best loved food. Some historians say he brought the plant with him from the Himalayan mountains and planted its seeds throughout India. Other tales say that Shiva himself created cannabis from his own body to purify the elixir of life, resulting in the epithet angaja or "body-born." It is believed that the word "ganja" originated from this term.

In the last of the four "books" of the Vedas, called the Atharva Veda, it is recommended to *take cannabis if you wished to commune with the Gods.* The Atharva Veda lists cannabis as one of five other sacred plants. You can find this in Book 11, Hymn 8 (or 6), Verse 15, where it says, "To the five kingdoms of the plants which Soma rules as Lord we speak. Darbha, **hemp**, barley, mighty power: may these deliver us from woe." According to *The Vedas*, a guardian angel lived in the cannabis plant's leaves.

And, according to *The Encyclopedia of Cultivated Plants*, Indians, holding that cannabis had spiritual qualities, used it to cleanse their sins, while Indian priests and holy men used cannabis to bring them to enlightenment. Cannabis helped them endure hunger, thirst, and pain.

Throughout Indian history, three types of cannabis formulations were—and still are—used for Hindu spiritual practices: bhang, which is a milky drink made from cannabis leaves and buds; *charas*, which is a type of hash made from resin; and *ganja*, which is the smoked flower. Consuming bhang cannabis milk to cleanse and purify the body during religious festivals is considered a holy act. Cannabis tea was a popular wedding beverage in India and a host would commonly offer cannabis tea to the guests who visited his home.

Bhang is still used in celebration among Indian families, especially during the festival of Holi. Holi festival marks the beginning of spring. The festival is a celebration of color, fertility, love, and the power of good over evil. For one joyful day and night each year during Holi, a large population in India celebrates with cannabis by making and drinking bhang. The drink contains nuts and spices, like almonds, pistachios, poppy seeds, pepper, ginger, and sugar. These are combined with cannabis and boiled with milk. I have included a recipe for Bhang at the end of this book, if you are interested in making it for yourself.

There are countless other stories about Shiva using bhang, burning ganja as incense, or smoking it from a slender, cone-shaped "chillum" pipe to find peace or inspiration.

Hindi holy men—known as "Sadhus"—to this day find enlightenment by combining the practice of yoga with the use of marijuana. Their belief system is primarily based on *The Vedas* and Yoga Sutras. According to the earliest texts of *The Vedas*, the Sadhus have been pairing charas—the hashish blend of cannabis, with their yoga practice since 2,000–1,400 BCE. The text also records Sadhus as drinking bhang for medical purposes.

The Yoga Sutras, compiled around 400 CE, outline the basic principles of yoga in 196 sutras, or threads. They are widely considered to be the authoritative text on yoga. In section 4:1 of the Sutras, the writers describe how self-realized beings exist on the earth and how one can attain this great realization. To paraphrase, this text illustrates the different ways one can achieve enlightenment: *"the subtler attainments come with birth or are attained through herbs, mantra, austerities of concentration."* This verse has been interpreted as spiritual realization coming from one or more of these things: 1) an exalted birth, 2) magical herbs, 3) mantras, 4) intense spiritual practice and absorption into Spirit. When I first saw this text, it astounded me that this wasn't common knowledge and that this wasn't being taught.

The Sutras were scribed by a sage described as compassionate and Buddha-like. His name was Sri Patanjali. He is widely considered by all yoga lineages as the father of yoga—all the different forms of yoga we practice today stem from his descriptive effort of what yoga is. According to historians, Pantanjali's aim in life was to end all suffering. He compiled the Yoga Sutras together to make ancient sacred teachings accessible to everyone. He wanted to end all suffering by helping humankind realize intrinsically who they really are.

Cannabis In Buddhism

As so do their Hindu neighbors, Buddhist practitioners in Tibet have a long tradition of using the cannabis herb for religious purposes. Gautama Buddha, the sage who established the religion of Buddhism in the 5th century BC, is believed by some to have lived on nothing else but one hemp seed per day on his path to enlightenment. There are also Buddha statues that depict him holding cannabis leaves. Certain Tibetan Buddhist sects believed the plant helped heighten awareness during ceremony and prayer and that it served as an aid during meditation.

Today there is debate among Buddhist practitioners over whether cannabis should be included in one's practice. Many point to the five precepts.

The *five precepts* are training rules undertaken by Buddhists across the world and have remained the same for thousands of years. The precepts were formed as a set of practices to protect the community and provide a guide for a life of mindfulness. The Fifth Precept is commonly translated as: *"I undertake the precept to refrain from intoxicating drinks and drugs which lead to carelessness."* Although in some direct translations, the Fifth Precept refers specifically and only to alcohol.

It is this fifth precept that causes debate in the Buddhist community about whether mind-expanding medicines have a place along a spiritual path. Despite the modern debate, there is proof certain Buddhist sects practiced the use of cannabis and other psychoactive plants. They are specifically prescribed for medicinal purposes in a text called the *Mahakala Tantras*. This sacred text is written from a varied group of Indian and Tibetan writers, which outline unique views and practices of the Buddhist tantra religious systems.

According to one article from the San Francisco Patient and Resource Center, Buddhists have used cannabis in tandem with meditation practices "as a means to stop the mind and enter into a state of profound stillness." The article states, "Various spiritual texts, including the Buddhist Tara Tantra, list cannabis as an important aide to meditation and spiritual practice."

Scythians and Cannabis

The Scythians were a nomadic people who traveled extensively around Europe, the Mediterranean, Central Asia, and Russia. They were expert horsemen, and one of the earliest people to use horse-drawn covered wagons. Scythians were known to use cannabis for religious purposes, and scholars credit them for spreading cannabis knowledge throughout the ancient world due to their nomadic nature.

The Greek historian Herodotus (484-425 BCE) wrote about the Scythians' use of cannabis in ceremonies to purify themselves after the death of their leaders.

Herodotus wrote that the Scythians would fix three tall wooden poles inclined towards each other and stretch woolen felts around them, creating a make-shift tent or teepee. They would place a dish inside the tent on the ground, put red-hot stones inside it, then throw hemp seeds onto the hot stones and inhale the vapor it created. "Immediately it smokes and gives out such a vapor as no Grecian vapor-bath can exceed," Herodotus wrote in *The Persian Wars*. "The Scyths, delighted, shout for joy, and this vapor serves them instead of a water-bath; for they never by any chance wash their bodies by water," he wrote.

Although this ritual was once thought to be myth, it was verified in 1929 when Professor S. I. Rudenko discovered a Scythian tomb near the Altai Mountains on the border of Siberia and Mongolia. In the tomb, he found the embalmed body of a man, a bronze cauldron filled with burnt marijuana seeds, as well as shirts woven from hemp fiber and metal censors for inhaling smoke that appeared for recreational purposes. Two gold bucket-shaped cups were also found in 2013 and are believed to be ancient bongs used by the Scythians. Inside them was a black substance that tested positive for opium and cannabis, which archaeologist Anton Gass believes were consumed simultaneously.

Cannabis in the Old Testament

Some history scholars and etymologists believe cannabis is mentioned several times in the Old Testament. In 1936, Polish etymologist Sula Benet proposed a new interpretation of the Old Testament. According to her, the Hebrew word "kaneh bosm" was mistranslated in the original Greek version of the Old Testament, which was written in the third century BCE, and the mistranslation has been repeated ever since. According to Benet, the Greeks mistranslated kaneh bosm to be the word calamus, a plant traditionally used to make fragrances, when in fact it referred to cannabis.

Kaneh bosm appears five times in the Old Testament—in the books of Exodus, the Song of Solomon, Isaiah, Jeremiah, and Ezekiel. The root word "kan" means "hemp" or "reed," while "bosm" means "aromatic."

The first mention of kaneh bosm in the Old Testament occurs with the prophet-shaman Moses, when God gives him instructions to create holy anointing oil, with kaneh bosm as an ingredient. In Exodus 30: 23-25, which dates back to 1446 BCE, God told Moses to create anointing oil with nine pounds of kaneh bosm, six quarts of olive oil, as well as essential extracts of myrrh, cinnamon, and cassia. In ceremonies, the oil would be poured over the head and body of a priest. If one believes the oil contained cannabis, it would then trigger psychoactive effects after soaking into the person's skin—those effects may have been perceived as a communion with God.

If it contained nine pounds of cannabis, the oil would certainly be potent and could explain the healing miracles of Jesus—since cannabis has been shown to be effective in treating many ailments, from skin diseases and glaucoma to multiple sclerosis.

In *The Origin of Consciousness in the Breakdown of the Bicameral Mind*, author Julian Jaynes suggests that ancient people were not as self-aware as modern humans, and so, when they were under the influence, may have perceived their own cognitive functions as voices from God. Benet also chronicles how the Israelites may have gotten knowledge of cannabis from the Scythians. Moses and his priests would burn incense and use holy ointment in a portable "tent of meeting," similar to how the Scythians also used tents for cannabis consumption.

Since the Scythians and the Israelites traded goods and knowledge, it makes sense to some historians that they would use the similar tent technique.

There *is* some scholarly doubt whether kaneh bosm actually refers to cannabis. Lytton John Musselman, author of *A Dictionary of Bible Plants*, argues that the plant *calamus* actually is capable of producing medicinal effects equal to those described in the Bible.

Rastafarianism and Cannabis

Rastafarianism is a social movement and religion created in the 1930s by Jamaican preacher Leonard Howell. Howell claimed Emperor Haile Selassie I of Ethiopia as the second coming of Jesus Christ, and that Africans were the chosen people and Ethiopia was their promised land.

Rastafarianism is very connected to cannabis. Rastafarians began incorporating marijuana (or "ganja") into their religious ceremonies in the late 1800s by indentured East Indians, who were brought to the Island to work after slavery ended. It just so happened that Jamaica had one of the best climates to grow the plant. However, Rastafarians condemn the use of cannabis simply to get high, as well as the use of other drugs, such as alcohol, tobacco, caffeine, heroin, or cocaine. These drugs are viewed as poison that defiles the body.

Rather than using cannabis just to get high, the plant is seen as a gateway to understanding. Cannabis is known as "wisdom weed" in the culture. Rastafarians believe that the "Tree of Life" mentioned in the Bible is in fact cannabis and that passages in the Bible promote its use.

These passages include: "He causeth the grass for the cattle, and herb for the services of man" (Psalm 104:14), "Thou shalt eat the herb of the field" (Genesis 3:18), "Eat every herb of the land" (Exodus 10:12), and "The herb is the healing of the nations" (Revelation 22:2).

Rastafarians consume cannabis in a ritual called "reasoning sessions." They commonly use a shared pipe called a chalice. It is passed around like a Christian communion cup. Reasoning sessions involve group meditation, and cannabis is thought to help individuals go into a trance-like state where they are closer to their inner spiritual self and God. Rastafarians refer to God by the name Jah.

Before the ceremonial cannabis is smoked, a short prayer is always recited: "Glory be to the father and to the maker of creation. As it was in the beginning is now and ever shall be World without end." Reasoning sessions are very important in Rastafarianism, as it is a time to debate how to live according to the Rastafarian outlook.

Weed Nuns

Cannabis is taking on a life of its own in modern times now that it is legal in Canada and multiple states in the U.S. One of the more prominent examples of a movement being formed around cannabis is The Sisters of the Valley. The Sisters are a group of women dressed as nuns who grow and sell cannabis while extolling its virtues. They have come to be known as the "weed nuns." The group was started in 2014 by Sister Kate, whose real name is Catherine Meeusen. In 2011, Sister Kate began calling herself a "nun" in response to the U.S. government calling pizza a vegetable. If the government could give pizza such a label, why couldn't she give herself a label as well? Sister Kate says that she didn't just call herself a nun out of protest towards the government, but as a nod toward nuns' history of activism in America, like during the civil rights movement.

Operating out of Merced County, California, nine "nuns" are employed, and the group produces mostly hemp with high cannabidiol (CBD) levels to be used for medicinal rather than recreational purposes. They also create balms, tinctures, oils, and soaps from the hemp. They create the products in strict adherence to the moon cycle, which they believe imbues healing powers. A ceremony for a new moon marks the beginning of a new production cycle, which lasts about two weeks.

The Sisters of the Valley model themselves after the Beguines, an ancient order of female healers from around 600 CE who lived communally and created herbal medicine.

Before joining the group, women take a vow to live simply, to have obedience to the moon cycle, and to be of service to the people.

Summation

As evidenced throughout history, cannabis has been intertwined in religion, ceremony, and the sacred. It has been used for its calming effects and its ability to help one reach higher mental ground. While some accounts of its use are contested, its natural prevalence and easy ability to grow makes it hard to discount its existence throughout humans' ancient and recent past. As legalization spreads around the world, new uses of the plant and beliefs surrounding it may continue to emerge—as people search for greater meaning and truth in the world.

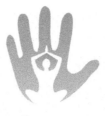

Chapter 3

TEACHING SACRED PLANT MEDICINE BEGINS

"You have to understand the purpose of life; the purpose of life is to do something which will live forever." —Yogi Bhajan

1. From the Personal to the Greater

Blending cannabis with yoga made me feel as though I was coming home. Tears would spring up when I was in a heart-opening pose—even when I had no reason to cry. The seeds of yoga knowledge that had been planted as long as 20 years earlier in my first yoga class began to sprout. The knowledge and wisdom grew roots in my being. I was blossoming in the teachings in a slow evolution that affected much more than postures and breathing.

I practiced yoga with cannabis once a week after that first breakthrough journey I experienced in Telluride, Colorado. The results of those weekly sessions spurred my desire to practice yoga and meditation daily— even without the plant medicine. The positive effects of combining cannabis and yoga, as well as the new and enhanced accessibility to the knowledge of my musculature and energetic systems stayed with me, even without the plant's influence. Once I was able to "see" the inner workings of my body, I could revisit that insight without being in an altered state of consciousness. I was in touch with what was going on inside and I realized, as both the yoga sages and the Bible teach, "The kingdom and queendom of heaven IS within you."

Rather than practice haphazardly, I made a routine of practicing first thing when I woke. It was cold in the mornings in the Colorado Rockies where I was at the time when I first combined cannabis and yoga, so I would sit in front of the fireplace in my fleece pajamas. All the teachings I had received from my wise yoga teachers flowed through me, giving me what I needed at the appropriate times. I would turn on soft chanting music by Snatam Kaur or Donna Delory, and start my practice by just sitting silently, letting myself feel every sensation I was experiencing in that exact moment. I wouldn't move until something in me needed more space or needed releasing. I decided to write down and record what I was doing and soon I began to understand that a design for a higher-level yoga class was coming through me...

It feels so good to stretch my legs out here and what if I draw my toes back towards my nose and now relax both feet. Oh my gosh, this is an actual pose. I've come into wide legged seated pose—Upavistha Konasasa. That's what this is supposed to feel like. Now I need to root my sit bones down. The mat feels grounding. This feels like I am rooting. I am growing roots. They are reaching through the mat and through the wood floor and into the foundation below, into the topsoil below and I am grounding. It's making me relax and I can let everything else go.

Could I teach this? I might be able to teach this. This is how I can teach this.

I realized I could put language to the dictates of this invisible current going through me. I knew I could describe the poses silently to myself and where I was going in my thoughts, so I decided to slow what I was doing way down, and let the practice teach me how to teach others.

As I moved slowly, I could feel the promptings in my body and translate those urges or needs into words I could write. This then would articulate the process of the flow that I was feeling. I was yoking my mind to my body and spirit. Moving carefully, staying in the pose as much as I could, I took up the pad and pen I kept near me and wrote: *Upavistha Konasana: legs are straight, relax your toes, all ten of them. Ankles are like taffy. Soften the calves and knee caps. Knee caps are like butter melting.*

I knew I could do it. This attentive practice with my body and mind were the very definition of yoga—Union. And I could write it all down.

The teachings of one of my most beloved and revered teachers, Erich Shiffman, came through the clearest. He had studied directly under three skilled and compassionate masters who brought yoga to the West: Jiddu Krishnamurti, BKS Iyengar, and TKV Desikachar. Erich taught the importance of feeling my body and flowing with what you felt inside. He taught that once you understood yoga postures or asanas as they are called, you move to the poses you are called to practice, but the important work is to take the practice of listening to your body with you through the day.

I never really got what he was teaching until now.

With the addition of plant medicine, Erich's teachings came alive in me. I knew what he was talking about. We have an inner teacher. We all have our own internal guidance system. If we learn to meditate and do yoga and simply pause occasionally throughout the day, we will feel the joy of "union with the infinite" more and more of the time. Cannabis was the great liberator within—to help me realize the intelligence in my cells and see the 'Yoga of Stillness' Erich taught.

As I practiced plant medicine more, a wise woman's lessons came through again and again. The teachings that showed up were from the author and metaphysical leader who I mentioned earlier, Louise Hay. Hay taught we create every so-called illness in our body through our thoughts. She taught how to use affirmations to change the thinking and heal the body. I'd hear her affirming words within myself when I was in certain poses.

While under the influence of cannabis, I had no doubt that thoughts do indeed create our reality, just as Louise taught—and that thought reality shows up first in our body. I started adding affirmations to my poses. For example, when I was lying on support blocks that opened my heart and throat, I would say something like, "I express myself freely and joyously." Or "There is plenty of love and I open my self to that love now and always. It is safe to keep my heart open."

My advanced yoga trainer from Scottsdale, Debra Garland, had taught me Kundalini yoga and pranayama (conscious breath) practices. These two disciplines or limbs of yoga—along with affirmations—shape the foundation of my morning practice. The plant medicine helps me feel and see the energy. Kundalini helps me transform it by using appropriate breathing, postures or kriyas (sets of energy exercises), while the affirmations heal mental patterns.

Before I used cannabis, these were all disjointed lessons that I learned intellectually and only knew in theory. But once I tried plant medicine, the different practices flowed together with broad results.

When I experienced the reverberating effects of this ordinary little morning practice carrying through into my daily life, I couldn't help but want to share it. People had begun asking why I seemed different, why I seemed more peaceful. One evening, back in Phoenix, I invited three friends over for cannabis yoga at my house. They wanted to each see what the combination would do for them.

Debra, Laura, Monica, and I sat in a circle around my coffee table. I had my chanting music playing. We started by each eating half a cannabis-infused gummy bear each. While we waited for the gummies to take effect, we set out blankets, blocks, and pillows. I pulled all the pillows off my two couches so we'd have every soft support we could want while we were in our poses.

Debra is my open-hearted neighbor. She has her medical marijuana card and uses plant medicine to help her sleep and to quiet her mind. She wants to explore inner realms. She knows a lot more about the plant than I do at this time. Monica, I met at a women's support meeting. I've known her for more than ten years. She is a mother of two like me and she is working a 12-step program. She is dedicated to healing any trauma she's experienced. She projects peace and loving kindness.

Then there's Laura. We had met at the gym where we were both into weight training. Laura is a sensitive. She feels everything! She rescues cats and is vegan. She graduated from veterinarian school, but never took the exam. She lost her mom recently and tells me she feels alone. She battles with alcohol abuse. I suspect she has deep trauma inside that has yet to come out. I feel grateful they are all with me and want to explore.

I begin. "Sisters, thank you so much for taking the time to explore this together with me. I'm so happy you are here. Here's what I am thinking we'll do. We will start by ringing the meditation bell and that will signal the beginning of this practice. We will give ourselves an hour and I will guide you into poses that help you feel and hear your body. When we are finished, I will ring the bell again."

"If there is a pose I can't do, what am I supposed to do instead?" Debra asks.

"Good point—always listen to you, to your heart and body! Not just in a yoga class, but as you go through your day. Ask yourself: *what might feel even better and more supportive for me in this moment* and then do that. You all know way more than a yoga teacher or anyone else what you need to do to take care of yourself." I see Laura letting out a long exhale. Her face relaxes.

"We will move in different poses. Use these pillows and blankets to make the pose absolutely supportive of you. I'll add some breathing suggestions throughout as I feel called to offer them. And then we will end with *savasana (corpse pose)*. I will ring the bell and then, if you'd like, we can set time aside for sharing about our experience. How's that sound?"

They all say, "Good."

We begin just as I had been practicing: we sit upright, close our eyes and feel everything in our bodies exactly as the sensations are. I call that aspect of the practice: *Landing*. We just look, just notice, without trying to change anything. And, I experience something new. Instead of tuning into only my body, I realize I can tune into all four of our bodies. It seems to me that when I focus on one friend, I can feel her interior states; when I tune into another, I can feel where she is coming from. I can feel what is going on with all of them. And I know that this is one of the latent powers coming from the plant.

I guide us to set an intention. After we take a moment for that, I direct them to pranayama to facilitate leaving the chattering mind and moving into the feeling space of their bodies. We do a series of different sustained poses, along with the breathing and affirmations I had practiced so many times on myself.

I do the poses in order of how the energy feels with the women. I do the poses that are coming to me that I feel their bodies need. I invite them to feel their connective tissues adhering to bone and of blood flowing in veins, and of lungs filing with air. I draw them deeper and deeper into their bodies through different poses and different pranayama (breathing techniques). We hold the poses long enough that they experience the real sensations of muscles unclenching and relaxing.

We move slowly and deliberately. Finally, it is time for *savasana* (corpse pose). They lie on their backs. I place lavender eye pillows over their eyes. Their arms are limp by their sides, palms facing up. Their legs are outstretched, and their soft feet fall away from each other. In my thinking, the yoga and cannabis have done their jobs. *Savasana* gives them time to feel what it's like to have unobstructed flow of blood and energy moving in our bodies.

I let them lie for a long time before I ring the chimes. The soft tones reverberate through the room. I invite them to bring their awareness back into their bodies and, when they are ready, I have them sit back up in a comfortable seated pose for our closing chant of Om. I can see their energetic bodies have opened.

As we finish, I invite the women to share their experiences. It is silent for a few minutes as each of them begins to integrate her experience. I can sense that all three women are in awe of the practice, at having been able to reach the place inside their bodies where peace lives all the time.

Laura and Monica had tears in their eyes. They try to explain the tears—they are tears of gratitude to be able to feel such deep letting go. What are they releasing? Only they could answer, but I suspect they are releasing emotional hurts, long standing resentments, and misunderstandings.

Laura shares first, "You know, I didn't do anything. I just breathed according to how you told us to and I got to this place where I merged with a lightness...and, you guys..." her voice breaks, "I got to see my Mom. She told me I can reach her anytime. All I need to do is breathe."

We all sit in silence for a while. Then Debra opens up, "It was a little scary at first to let go. But I followed the sound of your voice and it automatically happened. My body got soft and I've never been able to sit and touch my toes without bending my knees, but because you held us for so long I kept softening and softening until my legs straightened on their own."

I share how I can "see" inside their bodies when I focus on them individually and how at the same time, I can see my own interior state. None of us were expecting anything this dramatic. Certainly not me.

I bring out fruit I had prepared in advance and we nibble on that before they get ready to leave. As the talk winds down, we are filled with an overwhelming sense of peace that gathered there in my living room. The feeling of deep mutual respect lingers as we part ways for the night.

2. Taking the Practice to the People

After the gathering with my friends, I knew I needed to share this with more people. I had to. I went around to different yoga studios in Phoenix and, although most of the owners admitted to smoking marijuana regularly, they were afraid of the stigma and possible legal consequences attached to it. No yoga studio owners/teachers wanted to offer it in their places. I was about to give up hope and thought maybe I should just offer it in my home.

And that is when the owners from Urban Wellness, Patty and Doug Edgelow, said they believed in the physical and spiritual healing value of cannabis and yoga and would give the combination a go. Marijuana at that time in Arizona was only legal for medical purposes. You had to have a medical marijuana card to use it. I had gotten my card when I moved back to Arizona from Colorado. My medical condition? Anxiety.

In the beginning, I advertised the class by putting flyers in restaurants and on community bulletin boards. I limited the advertising so I could experiment with how the yoga flows went with different-sized groups.

My first Phoenix group came together on a Friday night. We met at four PM and partook at 4:20. We were a collection of very different people with one main thing in common. We all were open to the healing possibilities of cannabis and yoga. There was Phil. He was a machinist. He has long hair and is on the thin but toned side. He tells me he has inflammation and *candida*. He says he is changing his diet and dropping alcohol and instead is adding yoga and cannabis to his life. He said he had already lost 60 pounds. His family thought he was crazy because he no longer wanted to drink and was suddenly into yoga. It was causing friction with his wife.

Ivan also joined us. He is Hispanic, in his early thirties. He mostly remains quiet with the group. He is in deep pain after several back surgeries. He came to the classes to get greater flexibility and see if he could find pain release without pharmaceuticals.

Doug and Patty both attend the class regularly. Doug is a tall blond Scandinavian-looking Canadian in his 50s. He has a yoga practice already, but says he wanted to try this kind of yoga because he was looking for a deeper spiritual connection. Patty is also tall and lights up a room with her smile. She radiates kindness and is always making sure everyone in our group is doing okay. Several college students attend: Trevor and Dominique. They are friends and both have their medical marijuana cards. They are young and healthy. They just want to know how to tune into their bodies.

Elise also drops into class. I believe she has a shadow over her. My heart goes out to her. Her down-cast gaze tells me she is in emotional pain. Her nervousness is apparent. She confides to me privately that she has epilepsy and wants to try cannabis yoga to see if she can get off medications. She is studying to be a lawyer and the medications make her thinking fuzzy—which makes it impossible to concentrate. Another regular in the group is Linda, one of my closest friends. She is from Austria and, despite her busy, two-job schedule, makes it to almost every single one of our classes. She helps me set up and create a smoking area. She comes because the combination of cannabis and yoga lets her drop past her Austrian conditioning *and* her American conditioning and instead feel who she really is. We also have students who take the class without partaking in plant medicine at all. They say the yoga alone blisses them out. They say it feels like I am channeling the yoga. I get what they are saying, because this practice feels like that to me too.

I believe that what flows through me is a synthesis of kundalini, pranayama, asana, and affirmations. It flows in and through and out spontaneously. Cannabis smooths the flow. This new practice is unlike any yoga any of us have ever experienced. I imagine it is probably how yoga was practiced in the very beginning, thousands of years ago.

A stranger observing our work might judge us as a group of misfits. In fact, we were the beleaguered and the weary that had not given up on our trust in healing ourselves and seeing the beautiful in life despite the pain from past experiences. More than anything, I saw us all as courageous, spiritual warriors who said, "There's got to be a better way."

We were brave enough to try cannabis yoga despite the stigma and prejudices against marijuana—the beliefs that the plant was just for stoners and losers. There was plenty of research proving medicinal marijuana worked on a plethora of diseases, but in Phoenix, people still hadn't shaken off the years of vilification and misinformation surrounding the plant. At the time there was only limited research online that linked cannabis to yoga and spirituality. What I was aiming for with my students was not only the evidence for physical healings, which research proved was happening with the plant but, more importantly to me, spiritual healings. The medicine was helping us transcend our bodies and get to a place where we had direct contact with spirit. And it was in this place inside the physical experience that we were finding healing.

What these yogi brothers and sisters all had in common is they were looking for a better way to live without being anesthetized with pharmaceuticals, alcohol, or frantic activity and social media addiction. They were looking for a more intuitive way to exist in the modern human world without getting caught in its web of selfies and tweets and endless entertainment.

After our initial year of teaching in Arizona my husband and I found ourselves at a crossroad. The youngest of our six kids was graduating high school and we had always planned to move to Hawaii once that happened. But now I was torn. I felt like I was living my purpose and it was just coming into fruition.

My students and I knew we were on to something. That first year gave ample proof that the healing combination of cannabis and yoga flowing through us was real, not only for my own healing, but for the spiritual healing of others. My husband and I talked about what to do next. We decided to explore the option of creating Sacred Plant Medicine Yoga on Maui.

3. Bringing Sacred Plant Medicine Yoga to Maui

When we first arrived on the Island, I was surprised to discover that the cannabis laws were even stricter in Hawaii. People could get medical marijuana cards only if they had cancer, other major diseases, or had proof they suffered from PTSD. Under Hawaiian law, general anxiety wasn't reason enough to warrant a card. They did honor medical marijuana cards from other states and, because I had my card from Arizona, I was granted one in Hawaii.

Once we settled in the southern part of the Island, I again found myself on the hunt for a yoga space to teach. This time I didn't need to look far. The Wailea Healing Center was down the road from where we lived. We invited the owner, Rebecca Wilson, to dinner. She didn't know us, but graciously accepted the invitation. Brent explained what I had offered in Arizona and I shared my plans about what I wanted to do in Maui. She and her partner, David Connolly, talked over our proposal and welcomed us to their center with open arms. I had found Sacred Plant Medicine Yoga's first home in Hawaii.

I advertised the class in local spiritual magazines and posted flyers in organic grocery stores. I introduced my first class by offering a talk about cannabis and CBD combined with marijuana yoga. The studio was filled. People wanted to know more. They ranged in age from seventy to twenty-five. Most of them wanted to know how cannabis and CBD could help with their various ailments. But some were intrigued by how it could enhance their yoga and spiritual practice.

Those were the people that came back for my weekly class. These first students soon brought friends and family.

A yoga community centered on spiritual healing began to grow. Since that time, as of this writing, I now teach regularly on two sides of Maui. I teach in Wailea at the Wailea Healing Center; and in Haiku at The Temple of Peace, and I take this practice to neighboring islands for healing events and cannabis circles.

After a year and a half of teaching Sacred Plant Medicine Yoga, I felt called to add the cannabis element as an option to my life coaching offerings. Class after class, students would come up and say they felt so much release. Some would cry and tell me it was the most peace they'd felt in a long time. One woman said she had a huge breakthrough with a problem that had plagued her for a long time. Because of these living affirmations, it seemed natural to me to offer cannabis in conjunction with my life coaching that I currently did for clients. From there, we started conscious cannabis circles. These circles offer opportunities for group healings. People come together and mindfully partake in cannabis in a ceremonial circle and then lay on their mats and experience deep cannabis-assisted psychedelic inner journeys. The journeys can be very profound and elicit deep, deep healing of emotional, mental and even physical traumas.

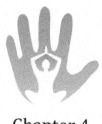

Chapter 4

OUR SPIRITUAL ALLY, SANTA MARIA

"We need enlightenment, not just individually but collectively, to save the planet. We need to awaken ourselves." —Thich Nhat Hahn

Waking Up

I open the sliding glass doors in the living-room and step outside. The grass is cool and wet. The dawn sky is sprinkled with the brightest stars. The growing sunlight creeps over the fragrant plumeria trees, pink bougainvillea and soft coral Frangipani. I watch the Pacific Ocean begin to shimmer.

This water of life reflects liquid sunshine. Myna birds call to each other. Sky and water seem to bless each other along the distant horizon. I experience this every morning when I sit for my practice. I sit outside on my white prayer rug on the grass in a comfortable seated position. A soft, cream-colored blanket wraps around my shoulders. I start my morning by sitting for at least 30 minutes. Then I start slowly stretching. As the morning warms up, so does my body through doing postures.

Each dawn I wake more. I feel my body, my thoughts, nature, and my unseen Spirit. Before I begin my meditation, I offer a prayer of gratitude that my brothers and sisters, the people I interact with every day, are also waking more. I pray we are being roused from our unconscious slumber. Then I sit on my white prayer rug and align myself with the gentle rousing.

I close my eyes for a moment so I can better feel the hum of life in the earth beneath and around me. My body IS my receiver. My skin houses my internal antennae and gives me the ability to tune in and receive. My morning practice connects me with myself, with my mother-Earth, and with the voices of my ancestors. As I adjust my spine in meditation; as I adjust my diet and what I let myself take in through my senses; as I clear toxins from my life and thinking: I learn how to better hear. And, having added Santa Maria to my practice, *I hear Hope.*

Author Stephen Gray powerfully describes the message I keep getting through Santa Maria (cannabis). In his book, *Returning to Sacred World: A Spiritual Toolkit for the Emerging Reality,* he teaches: "Learning to calm and silence the mind is the best way to learn to live well in this life. People build their whole lives on a narrative that involves almost constant thinking, but if you can be more present in life, moment by moment, second by second, you can experience a place of peace and groundedness."

For me, cannabis has amplified my other mindfulness practices and allowed me to transcend my constantly thinking mind and instead *feel* the present moment and *feel* what is happening in the now. Just by taking the time to notice what I'm feeling calms my heart. I feel my body deeply relax. I notice my body in each moment and I am present to it. This observance of what is happening right now becomes my spiritual practice. When I am that present to what is happening, my awareness expands past and through my body and I become connected to a larger whole.

Stephen Gray describes it this way—he says when you can reach this state, "you recognize that all is driven by love. You know who you are and you become an authentic presence, because you're not afraid of being your Self. You have the confidence to be who you are."

For me, once plant medicine began helping me release dross (dross is an accumulation of negative physical and energetic toxins that get stuck in the body), I became aware of an urgent message beyond my personal existence and well-being. I became very clear that we need to protect our planet. We need to protect the species on our planet. We need to protect all diversification of life including our own. As I continue to awaken, as I continue to remove limiting beliefs and social conditionings and return again and again to the truths I feel in my body, I become aware that I need to carry this healing, acceptance, and love directly to that which sustains us, our Mother The Earth. Again, author Gray best explains our spiritual predicament in this pivotal time of crisis and transformation. He writes that there are elders who say plant medicines are here now as key allies to help us heal ourselves and our planet. "Mystics and indigenous wisdom keepers are saying that an opening has now been created for a life-saving vision arising from and uniting all corners of the Earth. The vision tells us that to sustain our world we need to transcend dogmas, boundaries, and hesitation and awaken to our innate wisdom and our connectedness to each other, the living Earth, and the heart of the Great Spirit. It's up to all of us who 'get it' on some level to contribute to a saner, more sustainable planet, beginning with our own consciousness transformation and by natural extension our compassionate and creative engagement with the world."

Cannabis yoga dissolves a veil for me—and I hear this same message more clearly. Even without the plant medicine, many of us are hearing this message. There is an underlying sense of urgency. We, the people, have collectively gone asleep at the wheel. Most of us are in denial of what humans are doing to the planet and we are being distracted by issues that aren't important. According to numerous studies, books, and publications, including an article in *The Guardian*, human destruction of nature is rapidly eroding the world's capacity to provide food, water, and security to billions of people. Biodiversity loss is at the same crisis level as climate change. Some of the staggering findings are that exploitable fisheries in the world's most populated regions—the Asia-Pacific—are on course to decline to zero by 2048; that freshwater availability in the Americas has halved since the

1950s and that forty-two percent of land species in Europe have declined in the past decade. More than a third of land and three-quarters of freshwater resources are devoted to crops or livestock. Around 700 vertebrates have gone extinct in the past few centuries. Forty percent of amphibians and a third of coral species. If that current trend continues, sharks and marine mammals look set to follow.

Robert Watson, the chair of the Intergovernmental Science-Policy Platform on Biodiversity and Ecosystem Services (IPBES), which compiled the research says, "The time for action was yesterday or the day before... we must act to halt and reverse the unsustainable use of nature or risk not only for the future we want, but even the lives we currently lead."

My burning question has always been what kind of action can we take? How do we do that? What can you or I do that will make a difference? What will truly help? Many of us hear these grim reports and they seem bigger than what a person can handle. What can you or I do that will turn this trajectory around? How do I ensure that my five-year-old nephew Rudy gets to swim in the ocean with the Green Sea Turtles and that he can drink fresh water and breathe fresh air when he is my age?

In my burning desire to do something that makes some kind of difference - however small, I scoured the recommendations of leading environmentalists and compiled a list below. But above and beyond these suggestions I present, I sought deeper clarity and guidance. I took the time to listen. I stopped everything I was doing and took time to drop deep into abiding presence with the earth. I stopped looking at my phone, I stopped planning, I stopped writing this book. And instead one early morning, I packed a small bag with a jacket and some warm leggings, I threw in a bottle of water, nuts for snacking, and one of my husband's magic brownies. Then Yogi Bear, my Australian Shepherd, and I jumped into my jeep and drove deep into the heart of one of Maui's most treasured rain forests—the Makawao Forest Reserve. At 2,500 feet above sea level, the Makawao Forest Reserve features flowering ginger plants, towering, fragrant eucalyptus trees, and spectacular views of the island and ocean below. It's a bumpy winding road into the jungle. Once we get there, I pull into the gravel parking lot, shut the motor off and look around me. We are engulfed by ferns of all sizes including a variety of towering eucalyptus and pine trees.

I step out of the jeep and carefully unwrap the brownie. "Bom Shiva," I silently whisper before taking my first bite. The forest is enveloped in its own world. There is a hush broken only by swaying treetops and the occasional cardinal calling to another. I've done this many times before in different places and today is no different. I take off my shoes and put them in my backpack. Yogi and I begin our walk barefoot. We trek for hours up a looping path into the heart of this rain forest. When we finally stop, we find the perfect place to sit. It's on a dense blanket of leaves. Using my hands, I dig down through the underbrush and scoop rich, dark, fertile soil into my hands and lift it up to my nose, smelling its life. Then I sit in silence. The brownie is beginning to take effect. I am quiet for a long time. And I feel her. All of her. The trickle of water in a hidden nearby stream, the overhead swaying trees. The light breeze with a promise of rain on my face. The hum of crickets, bees, and moths. The chirping of unidentified birds. It all swirls together in one vibration. I can *feel* her pulse. I sit there in the forest with nature like you can sit with a child. I am simply *just* with her. It becomes clear what we need to do to save the planet...

The single biggest thing we *each* can do to save Mother Earth is to first stop. STOP! Stop everything and pay attention to her. Get outside. It doesn't matter if you live in suburbia or a city or the country. Find a place, perhaps under a tree where you can feel her. Go there and listen. Leave your phone at home. Get out of your head when you walk the earth. Be there. If it's possible, take your shoes off and feel her. Admire her trees, admire everything that is growing. Watch her sunsets and sunrises. Appreciate everything you can about her and all she offers. She is a living organism. (According to The Gaia hypothesis — The Earth's physical and biological processes are inextricably connected to form a self-regulating, essentially sentient, system.) Once you really see and hear her, the second thing you can do is see what she needs. What can you do from exactly where you are to help take care of your earth home? And the third thing you can do—move when you feel called in a direction. Take the action. Really do act—don't just think about it. Do it! Make it the priority. Your life depends on it. When our child is sick, we sit with her and we pay attention to what she might need so that we can help nurse her back to health. This is the same love we need to show our planet. And we start where we are. Pick up trash in your neighborhood. Join with a group of people who are planting trees. Ride your bike instead of driving. Stop using plastic of any kind, especially single use plastics. Love her. Show her love, concern and compassion and then extend that love to all living, sentient beings, wherever you are—all the time. To borrow the words from an old song— "What the world needs now is love, sweet love." It's true— that's how we save her. We love her. This is vital. Nothing else matters. I sat with her a long time that day and now it is a part of my weekly routine to visit with her there in the forest. I promised her I would do all I could to protect her.

Need a more comprehensive "to-do' list to get your creative juices flowing? Here are some simple and easily doable actions you can take that will make a big difference. As Gandhi said, "We have to be the change we are looking for."

1. Eat less meat. Why? Because raising animals for meat emits serious greenhouse gases and causes deforestation and water shortages that cripple the planet.

2. Plant trees. Why? Because they breathe in carbon dioxide and breathe out oxygen. Additionally, they provide habitats for birds and other wildlife. Trees trap CO_2 from the atmosphere and make carbohydrates that are used for plant growth. They give us oxygen in return.

3. Support the restoration of natural forests. Successful restoration enhances food security, improves our

air and water quality, and allows us to "weather" climate change better.

4. Use sun blocks when in the water that are coral reef safe. Why? Healthy coral reefs are one of the most valuable ecosystems on Earth. They provide billions of dollars in economic and environmental services, such as food and coastal protection. Keeping our oceans healthy is the same as keeping ourselves healthy. Even if you don't live near an ocean, chemicals in your everyday products end up in the ocean and in our water supply. Stop using chemicals that are not biodegradable.

5. Stop buying single-use plastics, like water bottles and plastic wrap and baggies. It can take up to thousands of years for plastic bags and Styrofoam containers to decompose. Which means we are going to be suffocating the planet, which means we could be suffocating our grandchildren if we keep using plastics. Plus, plastic contaminates our soil and water. The toxic chemicals used to manufacture plastic get transferred to animal tissue, and eventually enter the human food chain. Styrofoam products are toxic if ingested and can damage nervous systems, lungs, and reproductive organs.

6. Stop buying so many things period. It causes unnecessary wear and tear on the earth. When you buy a new kitchen appliance, for example, there's an environmental cost for the manufacturing process,

for the packaging, for the transportation, and for the marketing. According to more than one study, when you reduce how much you buy, you actually become happier and you help the environment! Try it! The time to act is now—before it is too late. It is time for us to recognize our connection to the earth, to all species and to all plants.

We are in a mutually dependent relationship with all life forms on the planet. Earth in turn provides everything we need. All plants offer immeasurable benefits to the earth. Since this book is about cannabis, let's take a closer look, for example, at the hemp plant or cannabis sativa plant. This is just one of many plants that feed our physical body and our spirit in many ways.

Hemp and marijuana are *different varieties* of the Cannabis Sativa species. The Hemp plant alone is remarkable in all that it offers us. It gives us food in the form of hemp oil and high protein hemp seeds and hemp flour; it's used for lotion, body oil, soap, cord or rope, and clothing. Hemp makes strong durable materials for home building and is used to make biodegradable plastics. Paper can be made from hemp more economically than from trees. Hemp can be made into fuel such as biodiesel. The petroleum industry has embraced the use of hemp in making its products. You can buy hemp products everywhere from Walmart to CVS pharmacy to Amazon. There's even a Bulk Hemp Warehouse which sells everything from hemp twine to kitchen towels, paper, food and pet supplies.

I believe that our plant allies are—at this time—calling out to us, just like the wisdom keepers are saying: "We need you. We need you to wake up. We need you to protect."

Many of us *are* waking up. We *are* coming to. We *are* beginning to quietly dismantle the frozen blocks of self. When we heal our own physical and emotional pain, the world can heal too. What happens within us is a microcosm of what is happening outside us in the world—the macrocosm.

Yogi Paramahansa Yogananda has said, "Change yourself and you have done your part in changing the world. People talk about doing big things, leaving a legacy, and making a difference in the world. But every extraordinary change comes from within you."

The Cree Indian Nation has a chilling prophecy it shares: "When all the trees have been cut down, when all the animals have been hunted, when all the waters are polluted, when all the air is unsafe to breathe, only then will you discover you cannot eat money."— It's not too late. All the trees have *not* been cut down; all the animals have *not* been hunted. Start now! Answer the call to live differently! There is time.

Sacred plant medicine can help us move forward, past blame into action. It illuminates the realization that we are all doing the best we can or we simply would have done better. There are many we could blame for the state of our world's predicament. Instead, let's use our energy to right the wrongs by starting with ourselves. We must now do the best *we* can.

Our ancestors and ancient mystics, environmental leaders, and now you and I know the way to save our planet.

We all know what we need to do to halt the loss of nature. The indigenous peoples of our land are still here with their ancient teachings. The Yogis and the masters have left instructions for us. It is not too late. We can re-member, meaning rejoin with our family of the earth by re-connecting with their truths. They teach that these truths are as close as our body. As close as our breath. When we feel our bodies, we can feel the earth. When each of us can feel our Self, we know what we need to do. It is as simple as that.

Yoga, meditation, and cannabis are three ways to get reconnected with our Self and our truths. There are many, many additional ways to return to the innocence of your truth. Find what works for you. Take the time to do whatever you need to do to get past your addictions, your limiting beliefs, and your self-sabotage so that you can really feel *you* again. When we are in touch with the truth of who we are (light inside a vehicle called a body) and the truth that we are all connected, we will no longer tolerate anything less than love for our Self and our planet. When we start to see that our body houses a sacred being of light, we treat our Self differently. With cannabis, these truths go from an intellectual knowing to a deeply experienced body knowledge.

It is crucial that I live according to *what I* feel. That means I have had to take concrete new actions that align with my need to protect the planet. In my and my husband's home, we eat mostly vegan, sometimes vegetarian, we practice turning off the water when we are brushing our teeth. We use candle lights at night and we use cold water to wash our clothes. We bike a lot and live where we can buy most of our food from the local farmers market. We use reusable cloth grocery bags and we've stopped the use of single-use plastics like saran wrap and zip lock baggies and plastic drinking bottles. To wrap our Christmas presents last year we decorated old saved brown paper grocery bags with markers. There is much more we can do. By staying open to our place on this Earth, we learn more every day.

Is the medicine calling for you to do things differently or is your own intelligence calling for you to do things differently? What are you doing already that takes better care of you and the Earth and your fellow/sister creatures? No one needs to know you are doing these things. This isn't about showing anyone how great you are or how much you care, this is about quietly making a difference in your tiny corner of the world. You know way more than anyone else what you can do and what you are being called to do. As C.S. Lewis said, "You can't go back and change the beginning, but you can start where you are and change the ending."

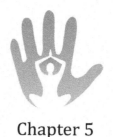

Chapter 5

HOW YOU MIGHT
EXPERIENCE A SACRED
PLANT MEDICINE CLASS

"What you are is what you have been. What you'll be is what you do now" —Buddha

You stand for a moment outside the Wailea Healing Center in Maui, Hawaii. The chants of ONG SO HUNG by Guru Singh waft through the open doors. Bird of Paradise, Bougainvillea, Night Blooming Jasmine, and shrubs a myriad shade of green surround this place of renewal and healing. It is peaceful here, and except for the chirps of birds, it is quiet. The west/ocean side of this center is all windows floor-to-ceiling, giving breath-taking views of the Pacific Ocean.

This center offers a refuge for those who seek alternative healing possibilities. Practitioners from varying disciplines rent out rooms to offer their specialties. When you walk through the doors you see a posted sign that says,

"Peace In." People usually pause to remove their shoes or flip-flops here. Once you step inside, you are in the yoga room. Delicate incense is usually burning in a far corner. The scents of frankincense and myrrh remind you that you have stepped into a place of peace. Sunlight streams in through the massive windows.

The teachers and healers here have studied and trained all over the world, but many of them feel as though some benevolent greater guidance drew them to Maui and the Wailea Healing Center. Monks and holy men and women drop in to share teachings and lectures. The regular practitioners offer massage, acupuncture, coaching, breath work, and sound healing. I guide Sacred Plant Medicine Yoga.

The center is located on the west side of Maui's volcano, Haleakala, which means "house of the sun." This volcano has, at twenty miles in circumference, one of the world's largest dormant volcanic craters. The ten-thousand-foot-high Haleakala has been quiet since 1790. Even though it has been asleep for centuries, invisible energy currents continue to flow from its shield crater.

This energy flow can't be seen, but it can be felt. I and many others have felt it. As rivers find the most direct course to the ocean, energy rising from the center of the earth through the volcano does the same thing. Once the energy reaches the top of Haleakala, it follows the same course a river would.

Magma and lava are not flowing down Haleakala at the present time, but when I pause and still myself, I can feel raw, clean, renewing energetic downdrafts coming out of the crater and flowing towards the ocean. This powerful downdraft once contained minerals made up from iron, magnesium, potassium, carbon, and more. Over time, these minerals eroded and dissolved, and then were reabsorbed into the soil. Now, it is just pranic energy that flows up from the crater center and is picked up by the wind at the volcano's surface and carried towards the sea. The Wailea Healing Center sits right in this blended path of earth and sea energy.

Besides the energy coming from Haleakala, there is another power source near the center. A Rainbow Eucalyptus Tree spreads its branches like a loving sentinel over the building. It stands forty feet high and its bark is all the colors of a rainbow: pink, blue, purple, yellow, and green. I have been taught that rainbows represent possibility. All the possibilities that are contained in the colors of the rainbow are being radiated up through the Rainbow Eucalyptus' roots and to its leaves. The tree's root system is directly under the foundation of the building. Its roots draw water and nutrients up to its trunk. They are converted to energy by the scientific miracle of photosynthesis.

I have felt this rainbow plant energy shower down from the tree's leaves, with blessings of possibility and renewal for everyone who is near. (Not everyone who comes to the Center sees this or feels this. Most people casually enter, concerned about whatever it is that is on their mind, but they may notice they are already feeling more peace, without even starting any kind of treatment.)

BREATHE

I meet my students at the door of the center, a little before 4 p.m. I have yoga mats set up in a circle with crystal healing bowls and lighted candles in the middle. Long time students greet each other in quiet, happy tones. They are women and men, young and old, all races, able bodied and disabled as well.

The students choose a mat and sit down. Most close their eyes and start bringing their attention to their bodies. Some quietly stretch while they wait for me to begin teaching. I slowly decrease the volume of the chanting music, "ONG SO HUNG," until there is no more sound except for the birds outside.

Those lying down, sit up. I wait for a minute or two until words want to be said through me. The words usually emerge something like this: "Welcome to Sacred Plant Medicine Yoga. It's beautiful to see you here. We come to this place and this space so that we can begin to feel and hear ourselves again. We create parentheses, if you will, around our lives for an hour, so that we can pause and feel and release anything that's not serving us.

"We will use different tools to help us with this releasing—pranayama —breath work, crystal bowl sound healing, essential oils, the ocean drum and chimes and sacred plant medicine in the form of cannabis.

"I'll take you through a journey into your body and guide you through different poses. As I do, always listen to yourself. You may become aware of something else your body wants to do or something you don't feel like doing. Please hear and do what your body is asking for. A yoga classroom is the perfect place to practice listening to yourself and giving yourself what *you* know you need. You know way more than anyone else what it is you need in your life.

"Drink lots of water as we go through the poses, that is one way we flush toxins and that which we don't need from the body. Make sure you are comfortable always. When we can let the body go soft, we stop clenching and that allows us to release holding patterns on a cellular level. That is true, not just in here, but when you step outside these doors. We practice and remember what it is like to stay soft in our body, so that we can live soft all the time and everything gets to just flow through us along with our breath."

I then ask the students if there is any part of his or her body that needs attention. Invariably, someone says, "my shoulders, or small of the back and hips." I make a mental note to start with one of those requests so we can get right to the parts of their body that are hurting the most. By this time, it's 4:20. I invite everyone to take out their pipes or vapes and we honor Santa Maria, the cannabis sativa plant, by giving it thanks before we take it in.

I say a prayer of gratitude for the earth and elements and cannabis sativa being a plant that is here to help us. When I am done, each of us brings their pipe or vape up to their forehead and says, "Bom Shiva" (Hail Shiva, Thank you, Lord Shiva) before taking a draw. We set our smoking devices down next to us and clear the mats of anything else we used to prepare our cannabis sacrament. When that is done, we are ready to begin asana. I ask everyone to meet me in a comfortable seated position on a yoga block or two.

I guide the students to close their eyes and straighten their spines. I then begin the process of taking them deeper into their body through their breath. "Where you are now, exactly how you are now, please exhale all the air out of your lungs, press your lips together and inhale in through the nose all the way to the top. When you reach the top, roll the shoulders back, sip in more air, close off the throat and hold. When you are prompted by your body—and take your sweet time—but when you are prompted by your body, turn your face to the right, open your mouth, and let it all go." We do this twice.

Now the students are softer. Now they are all a little more open. I bring in what I think is the most powerful part of the practice. The intention. I ask them to give themselves permission to let go of everything they've been doing up until this moment and everything they will be doing after our time together and instead give themselves permission to focus 100% on their selves and their bodies. I have them set their personal sankalpa (sankalpa is Sanskrit for an intention formed by the heart and mind—a solemn vow, determination, or will.) A sankalpa is a tool meant to harness the will, and to focus and harmonize the mind and body.

I slowly turn the music back up with a new soft song that helps us open and relax more. We start our series of poses, beginning with ones that target parts of the body the students requested. I teach the class through words and demonstrations, but I try to teach it in a descriptive way so that each student can keep their eyes closed if they wish through most of the class and, that way, concentrate on the sensations in their bodies.

I keep directing them to see in their minds' eye the inner parts of their body that we are working wit —so they know what they are doing and can stay present to where they are. An old yogi saying is, "Where our attention goes energy flows." And it's true, if the students are seeing or picturing the inside parts of their body they are working on, they are sending healing energy to that part.

For instance: when we are on our hands and knees in Table Top pose, I say, "Close your eyes and see your femur bone in the dish shaped socket of your hip. Like a wooden spoon, allow the thigh bone to scrape the inside of the dish. See that you are breaking up stuck matter that's accumulated simply because we always move in the same way. See that you are clearing and creating space in your hip. You are enhancing your ability to move forward more easily in your life. Your hip socket is the largest joint in your body and you are giving yourself greater mobility."

We continue working our way through the body, usually ending in a twisting stretch. My favorite twist allows renewing, healing energy to build and then spread in the body. We start by hugging the knees as close to our chest as possible, so we are almost curled up in a ball. Then, while keeping the knees as close to the body as we can, we let them fall all the way to the right, coming into a twist. We bring a bolster between our legs and relax there, keeping the ball. Then I have them reach left with their left arm and look left, while the knees still remain as close to the body twisting right.

"We are compressing your digestive organs—placing them under weight. This constricts circulation. When you release your twist, there will be a rush of fresh blood in your digestive organs. Fresh blood flow equals fresh oxygen and nutrients. You are enhancing your ability to not only digest your food, but your life."

We use props in every class: cushions to lie on in certain poses and foam blocks to support us in various poses. Sometimes I pull light sandbags out and put that on people's lower back when they are in Child's Pose. Throughout the poses, when I am internally directed, I offer instructions for different pranayama (breath exercises). If the students' collective energy feels unfocused and they can't seem to drop in as easily, I employ breath retention types of pranayama. If they are focused and totally with me, I call in lighter pranayama exercises so they can more easily access the subtle energies inside their body.

We also use mudras, ancient hand gestures that call and lock in deeper energies. Mudra is Sanskrit for the word "seal." Buddhist and Hindu teachings say the position of our hands has the ability to influence the energies of our physical, emotional, and spiritual body. Mudras help link the brain to the body, soothe pain, stimulate endorphins, change the mood and increase our vitality. If we practice the mudras, the minute we take a particular gesture on, we are strengthened in an alignment of all that the mudra signifies.

For example, Gyan mudra is the classic meditator mudra you see in most pictures of people meditating. The pointer finger presses into the thumb and the three remaining fingers extend straight (very similar to the okay sign we make with our finger and thumb). Hands in prayer are another mudra.

(Anjali Mudra) Prayer hands say so much more than words can convey. When our hands are in prayer, palm to palm, we are recirculating and building internal energy. Most people think Anjali Mudra is a form of salutation to another, which it is, but most importantly, it is us recognizing and honoring our own interior truth and light and regenerating that light. This mudra ends up becoming a healing directive to oneself, not just a greeting to another. As with all mudras, it's silently communicated to and through the entire body.

When the students are in certain poses, I will also use plant medicine in the form of essential oils and infusions to further enhance the students' abilities to use their senses *to come back to their senses.*

After an hour of movement, we end our series of postures with savasana—corpse pose, where everyone lies down on their backs with their legs slightly parted, feet falling away from each other and arms away from their body. Some choose to put bolsters under their knees, so the pose feels really nice on the lower back. I place chilled lavender-scented towels over each student's eyes. I play crystal healing bowls which emanate sound vibrations that wash over all of us. I use the ocean drum, which to me, feels like rain washing my cells. Sometimes I use chimes and rattles along with music to deepen their ability to merge with the feeling of lightness and air. We then rest for at least five minutes, usually it's fifteen.

When they're rested, I then guide them to bring their awareness back into the room, back into their body. I ask them to keep their gaze internal as we move into a circle to chant a closing OM. I always let everyone know if they ever feel like they cannot drive after this experience, that we will get them a ride, either through Uber or a friend. (For many of the newcomers, this is the first time they have fully allowed themselves to breathe deeply and that, with the cannabis, can make them a little-lightheaded.)

The students wipe their mats, collect their belongings, and hug each other. They hug me. I can clearly see almost everyone in the class is breathing more calmly. Invariably someone, usually a newcomer, will come up and tell me they feel huge release, as though something dark and heavy has left their body.

One by one, everyone slowly leaves. They walk out the door with the sign on the inside that says, "Peace Out" on it. They take the three steps down to the sidewalk and pass under the Rainbow Eucalyptus Tree. They walk down the hill to the parking lot, while the invisible flow of Haleakala's healing energy continues to course through their path and through them.

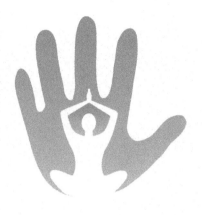

PART 2

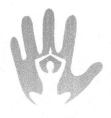

Chapter 6

THE EIGHT LIMBS
OF YOGA

---

*"Yoga is the journey of the self, through the self,
to the self." —The Bhagavad Gita*

To understand where this practice can take you, it's important to include an overview of the most fundamental foundation of yoga, which is The Eight Limbs of Yoga, as found in the *Yoga Sutras*. Practicing Sacred Plant Medicine Yoga automatically intersects this ancient pathway towards profound teachings and leads us by the hand through different bodies of knowledge. The plant medicine brings us to the Eight Limbs of Yoga whether you possess an intellectual knowledge of them or not. If you embark on this Plant Medicine Yoga journey, it will serve you to have an understanding of where you are going and what you are seeing and experiencing. When you listen to your body and give it full permission to express however it needs to, you may spontaneously start doing poses you've never been taught before or breathing exercises you had no training in. You may also begin to see glimpses of your different energy bodies that reside inside and outside of your physical body. This practice allows you to experience and see first-hand what the ancients were trying to teach. When you can "see" into the mechanics of your body, you will be able to see what you need to do to heal stagnation in different areas. These limbs or 'bodies of knowledge' can show you how to read energy. And it is all energy!

As I briefly mentioned in chapter two, The *Yoga Sutras* were compiled and organized 1,700 years ago by a man named Sri Patanjali. Pata (meaning leaves) and anjali is the mudra of the hands together in prayer. Patanjali was an ancient scholar and his goal, just like the Buddha's, was to end suffering. In the *Yoga Sutras*, he gathered early philosophical teachings, such as the *Upanishads,* and then he added spiritual practices, which elevated the teachings from mere philosophy to a practice people could actually experience. Patanjali saw that if people could develop physical and spiritual disciplines through yoga and meditation their suffering would be relieved. The *Yoga Sutras* and eight limbs outline how yoga—as a way of life, can help people bring peace to their own mind and show them how to live connected to a flowing source of vitality, ease, and union with all things. Patanjali knew that, if each person was free of suffering then the world would be free from suffering as well.The Sutras are a series of 196 aphorisms that were originally strung together and taught through singing. Sutra means thread in Sanskrit. The teachings were memorized and handed down thread by thread, or song by song, from generation to generation for thousands of years before Patanjali organized and wrote them out. This ancient foundational text defines the practice of living your yoga— which goes way beyond mere yoga poses. The first two limbs are called the Yamas (abstinences) and the Niyamas (observances). They outline moral principles and observances that prepare a practitioner for the profound inner work and higher energy to come. Here are The Eight Limbs spelled out:

1. The Yamas - Ethical considerations to help guide your interactions with others.

2. The Niyamas - Practices that have to do with self-discipline and world views.

3. Asana - Physical postures practiced in yoga. This is where Sacred Plant Medicine Yoga first falls into the eight limbs. But as I mentioned earlier, plant medicine will also bring you back and around to the first two limbs as you continue observing and practicing your yoga.

4. Pranayama - Breath Practices.

5. Pratyahara - Withdrawal of the senses.

6. Dharana - The practice of intense concentration.

7. Dhyana - The state of being keenly aware, without focus.

8. Samadhi - The state of ecstasy— through connection with the divine.

This eight-fold path is written in a divine order. When we practice Sacred Plant Medicine Yoga, we embark at "asana" and flow naturally on this unfolding path through the rest of the limbs. Assuming you are already practicing the Yamas and Niyamas —which boils down to living a good, moral life based on honesty and doing the right thing for all sentient beings—then practicing postures with Sacred Plant Medicine Yoga naturally leads to the next step: to an awareness of how you are breathing (this next limb is Pranayama). Each limb could be explored and practiced for a lifetime. Once understood and practiced, the limbs overlap and intertwine often. There are so many levels of knowledge contained within each of the limbs. For example, there are so many variations of breathing styles contained within the mindful practice of inhaling and exhaling. In fact, you will learn that different breathing styles bring you to different levels of consciousness. On to Pratyahara, there are so many methods and ways to withdraw the five senses which then make you acutely aware of your own interior space. This then can lead to development of your sixth or intuitive sense.

To summarize, doing asana makes you aware of how you are breathing while you are holding a pose. This then makes you aware of how you are breathing in and outside of a yoga classroom. Once you realize you can bring fluidity to your breath in all your affairs—on and off the mat—you become aware that breath work can help you reach different levels of consciousness. This then leads you to the next limb: Pratyahara and then Dharana—deeper concentration; which takes you to Dhyana, a state of supreme awareness of subtle energies, which brings you to Samadhi—merging with "All That Is."

I find the more I learn, the more knowledge unfolds, making me realize I know so little. The purpose of this knowing is exactly how Patanjali saw it. It's to simply help us live fully with a deep sense of ease, peace, and wellbeing, no matter what is going on around us. This is one way we are the "peace we wish to see in the world." As you follow the path of Sacred Plant Medicine Yoga, you may see you inadvertently have become a peace activist.

When yoga is practiced over a period of time, we are able to release anxious, life-draining or trauma-filled energies from the body. This helps keep us clean and clear toxicities of all kinds: toxic thoughts, toxic foods, toxic people, bad air, etc. When we are clearer in our mind and in our body, we have space to more readily absorb the finer, higher subtle life-giving energies called Prana. This allows us to then receive pure transmission from on high. We become an open vessel capable of receiving direct enlivening transmission of the One Spirit. This is the practice of a lifestyle. Observing the eight limbs as you practice Sacred Plant Medicine Yoga is how we live our yoga. The best book I have found for easier to understand translations of the Yoga Sutras is called *Inside the Yoga Sutras* by Reverend Jaganath Carrera. I highly recommend using it and studying it as a guide for living your yoga.

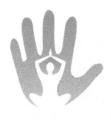

Chapter 7

THE IMPORTANCE OF SETTING AN INTENTION

"Awakened doing is when you don't create suffering anymore for others—or for yourself—by your own actions. It also implies that your primary intention, the focus of your attention, is on the "doing" in the present moment, rather than the result that you want to achieve through it." —Eckhart Tolle

When we open ourselves to the mysteries of the unseen, we open ourselves to bodies of energy that are invisible—but real. It is wise, prudent, and I think absolutely necessary to set intentions before communing with Santa Maria. And I absolutely recommend that everyone set an intention before embarking on a voyage into the unseen—with or without Santa Maria.

Intentions in and of themselves are an energy. So, we use the intention as a way to step into the invisible and remain guided along the current we have decided we want to play in.

In the words of another one of my beloved teachers, Kamani Desai, "Intention guides us on our journey in ways a goal cannot, making every step of the way both a direction and an endpoint simultaneously. In the perpetually unfolding journey of spiritual growth, the power of integrative intention opens the door to witness of our thoughts, emotions, and actions through good times and bad. When understood in its depth and potential, intention empowers us to direct our lives and our spiritual growth. It is the rudder that steers our 'ship' on its true course through both calm and tumultuous waters." An intention is not a casual matter. This is not a simple little wish. An intention is the guiding influence or focus that delivers to us, in the highest way, that which we say we want to experience or gain clarity on. The intention keeps us present while we experience what's in front of us.

When cannabis and intentions are combined the results of meditation are amplified. Santa Maria infuses your intention with greater power.

Setting an intention before you meditate, do yoga or any other activity gives you space to determine your mindset, which affects the caliber of integrity you bring to what you are about to do. Take this time before partaking of the Sacred Plant Medicine to align with those energies that match your intent. Then when you commune with Santa Maria you can more easily see and feel your intention manifesting.

When you don't take time to set your intention you subject yourself to a possible meandering, unfocused experience. Intention-setting provides a road map or a personal guide, if you will, to what you are looking for. For example, if you want to go to New York from California and you just got in the car and started driving, you could get lost. Your trip could go on for months. But if you used a map, you would be guided there more efficiently, and you would know where you are in the journey. Intentions are like the map, except they carry you more than guide you, to whatever you want.

When we don't set an intention, whatever we are already randomly thinking about or what is dominant in the subconscious is magnified. When you harness an intention and then have communion with the medicine, cannabis becomes your ally for something as simple as relaxation or as deep as enlightenment.

I believe that what we think about is what we create more of. We are the creators of either our heaven on earth or our hell on earth. That is why chanting mantras are so powerful. That is why saying prayers are so powerful. Our thoughts are just like intentions. Our thoughts either raise our frequency or lower it.

When we set an intention, we align ourselves energetically to a frequency that is always there, but not necessarily in our conscious experience. The act of intention-setting situates us on a level or experience that has the potential to guide us towards healing and expansion or its opposite—destruction. Intention-setting is just getting clear on what we want to bring in to our experience. My dominant intention most of the time is to feel connection to Source 24/7.

Everything we practice in a Sacred Plant Medicine yoga class is done to support us in being more mindful during the class and after. More heartful. More body-full. We practice tuning into what we are feeling in our body in class, so that we remember to feel our body while we go through our day.

Being aware of what our body feels like, where we are now, keeps us aware of the present moment. When we know what it feels like to be present, we more quickly realize when we've gotten lost in our thoughts and can bring ourselves back to feeling. The more we practice staying present in a simple little yoga class, the more mindful and awake we remain in each moment outside of class.

We want to live mindfully with awareness, fully awake to what is in front of us in each moment. That is when we are truly alive. We learn to breathe while we are in difficult poses to help us remember to breathe when we are in difficult life situations. When we are conscious of our breathing, we are conscious of the present moment.

It is the same with setting an intention. We mentally align with that which we are seeking, and we automatically step into its current through our desire. We stay in that current through our breath. That is why setting an intention is of the utmost importance. Intentions help us create and experience the life we dream of. If we don't get conscious of what we want to experience and intend, then old thought programming runs us. If we think the same old thoughts out of habit, we will experience the same life, over and over again.

When I'm teaching a class and suggest we set an intention for our practice, I usually say something like: "I invite you to set an intention for the next 60 minutes. Maybe it is something you'd like to experience more of, maybe it is something you'd like to let go of. Whatever you wish, I invite you to silently say to yourself for the next 60 minutes, I intend to...."

They fill in the blank on their own. While they are doing that, I do the same thing for me. I tune into my body and feel it. Then I sense the energy of the class and I sense what is needed. Once I've tuned into the class, I set my intention according to what I feel the class needs, so perhaps my personal intention is to "listen." I will tune into them, simultaneously listen for guidance, and listen to my own body. Maybe the energy from the class that day feels heavy, in which case, my intention would be to reflect and magnify their love and light.

The best explanation for the power of intention is to see it as analogous to the power of prayer. I can't explain how prayer works, just as I can't scientifically explain the way electricity illuminates a light bulb. But when I switch the light to on, it turns on through the current of energy that flows to the bulb. This is exactly what happens when we set an intention. An energy current creates the manifestation of whatever it is we are intending.

When we can look at our physical body as a sophisticated, cosmically designed vehicle that's evolved over time to receive information on many different levels, we see we can receive sensory input as well as non-sensory impressions. We can receive thoughts and we can send thoughts. We might not be precisely aware of what other people are thinking, but we all have experienced, at one time or another, a "vibe" when we are around a person or certain people. That "vibe" can be felt whether or not words, looks, or glances have been exchanged. We can simply *feel* it.

On a bigger and deeper level, when we take the time to set an intention, we cast out to the universe our desire to receive a certain flow of energy that creates a measurable change in our experience. The best way to test this theory is to experiment with it on yourself. Your intelligence and experience are your best guides. Get clear on what you want to intend and then declare it silently or out loud in an actual declarative positive sentence. For example: My intention this morning is to feel peace and joy. Or, for the rest of this day I intend to see the best in everyone. I intend to be present and listen. Take the time to declare what you want to experience and then go forward from this declaration knowing it is happening as you have stated.

Segment Intending is something I've practiced for years with positive results. I learned it from author and medium Esther Hicks, who channels a group of entities called Abraham. Abraham teaches how to make sections or segments of our day and create intentions according to the circumstances we want to experience in each section.

For example, when we wake up in the morning before getting out of bed, we would set our first intention. Let's say it is to have a beautiful day filled with love, health, peace, calm, and presence. Then, when we eat our breakfast, we set another intention. Perhaps this one would be to receive full nutrition and vitality from the food we are eating. When we get in our car to drive to work, we would set another intention. "I intend to enjoy this drive and see the beauty around me. I intend to arrive safely, feeling greater peace and feeling refreshed." Then before we walk into our work building, we would set another intention. "I intend to be the center of calm and peace. I intend to see the best in everyone around me. I move through the office filled with love and light."

This might sound like a lot of work to you. It's not. We are thinking all the time anyway. Why not use that gift? And, instead of reacting negatively to life as it happens to us, as if we are continually being victimized, we get to see differently. Intentions help us see anew.

For example, before you start driving, let's say you have set the intention to enjoy your drive, using the affirmation above. Now when you are driving, instead of getting irate at the driver that threatens to cut you off, you drive safely and enjoy the beauty of the passing scenery. If a driver does cut you off, it's incidental. You no longer give attention to that. Who cares? You will be so busy enjoying the beauty around you that the other driver's rudeness is no longer a factor. As you practice this, you may find that slowly but surely, fewer drivers actually try to cut you off.

Author and visionary Paul Cuelo says, "When you really want something to happen, the whole universe conspires so that your wish comes true." The Bible says, "Pray without ceasing." That is what we are doing when we set intentions. That is what we are doing when we practice saying affirmations as well. We are bringing mindfulness to where we are in the moment. My teacher, Paramahansa Yogananada, said, "Never think that God does not answer your prayers. Every word you have whispered to Him He has written in His heart, and someday He will answer you." We are always creating through thought, so being aware of what we are thinking about and directing those thoughts can create a life by design, rather than by default. The channeled entity Abraham says the same thing in a more contemporary way, "Your prayer causes you to focus and the law of attraction causes everything in the universe that's in vibrational harmony with your focus to come to you." Experiment with setting intentions for a month if this resonates with you and see what it does.

More importantly, please set an intention before you commune with Santa Maria. She will be there as an invisible friend to help you along your path of spiritual growth. And, your intention shows respect—for her and for your self.

Here is A Simple Way to Set an Intention Before Partaking in Sacred Plant Medicine:

1. Get quiet.

2. Ask yourself what you would like to experience more of or to let go of.

3. State it in a declarative sentence, silently or out loud. "For the next (thirty minutes or hour or whatever amount of time you want), I intend to _____ (fill in the blank with what you desire, i.e., "be present,"

"hear the messages from my body," "experience connection." Or "for the next sixty minutes I intend to let go of everything and anything that gets in the way of feeling myself fully."

With practice, setting intentions regularly for yourself can become a powerfully loving habit. It can help you regularly check in with yourself and stay true to the best that is in you.

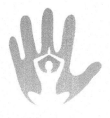

Chapter 8

CREATING YOUR OWN AT-HOME SACRED PLANT MEDICINE YOGA PRACTICE

"Whatever is fluid, soft, and yielding will overcome whatever is rigid and hard. What is soft is strong." —Lao Tzu

When you create a yoga practice that you can consistently engage in, you exponentially increase your ability to connect with your true self or the Divine or whatever you would like to call Source. To begin with, ask yourself how many times a week you can do your yoga? Where can you create space for this in your life? I don't want to ask what your schedule allows, because we can all find reasons to be busy. Instead, I ask what will you give yourself? How many times a week can you sustainably give yourself private movement? I practice my private yoga with sacred plant medicine once a week. But I do yoga every day, but not

111

always with the medicine. It's important to find a schedule you can honor because it strengthens your concentration. And that simply means you have access to greater wells of peace. Give yourself as much private yoga as you can, but make sure it doesn't add stress to your "to-do" list.

Sri Dharma Mittra said, "Move your joints every day. You have to find your own tricks. Bury your mind deep in your heart, and watch the body move by itself." See what amount of yoga feels good for you and honor it.

Maybe in the beginning you do your private marijuana yoga practice once a week. The more you practice the easier it is to drop into your body the minute you sit down. Once you test out and then establish a routine, you can keep adjusting your practice according to what your nervous system can handle. We each have to find balance within us that works with the medicine and our outside responsibilities. Right now, I find once a week partaking in my own private yoga ceremony keeps me connected to flowing source and then I practice what I learned the rest of the week without the medicine. Invariably I teach what I am practicing in my public classes and I implement and integrate that in my life.

Here is a framework for private plant medicine yoga you can follow if you wish. This can augment your ability to reach a deeper part of yourself, which can transmit through your body. I'll number the order in which I do this down below, but first I will explain what I do and why I do it.

I get my favorite faux lambskin rug and set it outside on the grass at sunrise. I have my mala beads on. I set my timer on my phone, so my monkey mind doesn't have to wonder how long I've been sitting. I sit and get comfortable. Then I partake. I draw in only one inhale. Less medicine is better for me. Next, I pray. I pray for forgiveness. I pray to feel, I pray for my family and friends. I pray to connect to the teachings of my ancient masters and the teachings from the plant. I say the Lord's Prayer: *Our Father who art in heaven, hallowed be thy name. Thy kingdom come, thy will be done, on earth as it is in heaven. Give us this day our daily bread, and forgive us our trespasses, as we forgive those who trespass against us. Lead us not into temptation, but deliver us from evil. For thine is the kingdom, the power and the glory forever and ever. Amen.*

Then I say the third step prayer from Alcoholics Anonymous: *God, I offer myself to Thee—to build with me and to do with me as Thou wilt. Relieve me of the bondage of self, that I may better do Thy will. Take away my difficulties, that victory over them may bear witness to those I would help of Thy Power, Thy Love, and Thy Way of Life. May I do Thy will always.*

Next, I pray to my guru Paramahansa Yogananda and his lineage and to Neem Karoli Baba and to Jesus Christ. I find myself praying for forgiveness because invariably when I first partake, I become aware of fragments of judgments that have accumulated in me, fragments of conditioning and projections I put on people. I'm not aware I'm judging when I do it. It seems minor but judging people and categorizing them and labeling them adds physical sludge to our body. It blocks the flow of prana in and around me. Energetically it makes me forget that we are all beings of light in a body and we all have important work to do.

I then set my intention (which we covered in the previous chapter). My intention starts by saying to myself, "*I give myself permission to let go of everything I've been doing up until this moment. I give myself permission to let go of everything I am going to be doing after this session. Instead, I bring my attention and my focus one hundred percent on me and my body. My intention for the next hour is ____.*" And I let myself feel what I need and I silently state it.

Once this is done, I sit still until I feel the need to move. I keep my notebook by my side so I can jot down the movements that come to me as I flow into them.

Here are suggested steps for your practice:

1. Find a special private place you can dedicate to your meditation and yoga practice.

2. Take the plant medicine in with reverence. Be aware it will help you move into other states of consciousness.

3. Pray for forgiveness, pray for help in concentrating, pray to feel connection.

4. Set your intention.

5. Sit in stillness and let your body become soft.

6. Let your spine elongate so that your heart shadows over your hips and your throat shadows over your heart.

7. Let every muscle soften while your spine stays lifted.

8. Wait until you are prompted by your body to move.

9. Then give your body what it's asking for. Maybe you feel like you want to fold forward, maybe you will feel like your neck wants to stretch, so you do head rolls. You will know what your body needs to do by taking the time to feel it.

10. When you do move, concentrate on picturing your muscles, joints, connective tissue and fascia. Picture the inside of your body as you respond to how it wants to stretch and move.

11. When you feel complete, thank yourself for taking the time to really tune in and listen to yourself!

The more you tune into your body while you are practicing your sacred plant medicine yoga, the more you will be aware of your body while you move through your day-to-day activities. Body awareness empowers and enlivens everything you do. You will grow in consciousness and awareness. And that awareness will slowly expand past the confines of your skin. You will become more aware of everything in you and around you. When you approach your life from this place of greater understanding, you will have better mastery over your emotions, thoughts, and reactions. And you will be present to the reality of what is happening in the moment.

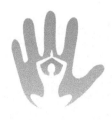

Chapter 9

CANNABIS-ENHANCED MEDITATION—COMMUNING WITH THE DIVINE

"You should sit in meditation twenty minutes a day, unless you are too busy; then you should sit for an hour" —Old Zen saying

Your Meditation Practice

The most powerful aspect of Practicing Sacred Plant Medicine Yoga may be where this practice takes you. Sacred Plant Medicine Yoga is a natural primer for meditation. It can be a guide that leads you deep into the wonders of the universe as explored through your body.

It doesn't matter what meditation style you embrace. I encourage you to try different ones until you find one you completely resonate with. It doesn't need to feel like work— or yet another responsibility. Meditation is your gift to yourself—and your world.

Meditation is a practice, so give yourself time to be with different practices for a while, spending at least a full month with an individual technique before you try a different one.

For me, the most incredible thing about meditation is it can bring me to a *felt* realization of Divine Being, the physical knowing of an omnipresent, omniscient, all-pervading essence that flows through all things, *all* things—including me. This felt knowing surpasses all thinking, theorizing, debating, and religious dogma. It allows us to *feel* Presence as clearly as I can feel my leg pressing against the leg of the table I am sitting at right now as I write this chapter.

I do Sacred Plant Medicine yoga because it feels so good in my body; it clears me of dross and calms the fluctuations of my mind, so that I move/am moved toward a place of ease and grace. Once I am calm and peaceful, I am quiet enough to feel the subtle energy of spirit. If I practice coming to this place regularly enough, then I can transcend my physical environment by withdrawing my senses and bringing concentration to The Being, which allows me to merge more often with the *All That Is*. We *can* feel the bliss of supreme connection to Spirit here. Now. Not in some far-away heaven or time.

I can only share what I practice—what I truly know. If these meditation practices call to you, then great. If not, there are many different styles of meditation, so please explore until you find one that makes you feel like you can grow with it. As for the ones I'm introducing here, I've included background information and deeper descriptions of how each practice originated and what they mean.

There are countless ways to meditate. Over the years, I found several pure meditation techniques that work for me. They come from two different spiritual traditions: Buddhist and Hindu. Although from different traditions, each teaching is true to its roots.

I chose sitting meditation styles that resonated with me. They are easy and light. I practice at least one of them every day. There is The Relaxation Response, which is similar to Transcendental Meditation (T.M.). It is the first meditation style I learned when I was fifteen. I also practice Hong Sau meditation as offered by the Self-Realization Fellowship, under the teachings of my Guru Paramahansa Yogananda. My third practice is Vipassana Meditation. Again, I recommend you try one technique for at least a month before moving on to a different technique.

All of these meditations can be more powerful if you create a space in your home that's just for meditation. It doesn't have to be fancy. It just needs to be a spot you can come to regularly where you will not be interrupted—so you can concentrate fully. If you wish to create an altar or bring in objects that call in and represent higher vibrations for you...do so. I meditate with Mala beads. If I meditate inside I do it in front of my altar, on which I've placed pictures of great saints, gurus, heart-shaped coral pieces, crystals and candles I've received over the years. But the first place I ever meditated regularly was in my bedroom closet. It was the only place in my childhood home where I thought I could be alone. I shared a bedroom with my sister.

The second most important factor is to observe a regular practice, as regular as drinking water. You need to drink water consistently and daily so that you get the hydration your body needs. With meditation, you need to do it daily and regularly so that you can strengthen your ability to tune in and connect. The practice of meditation is practicing the art of *fine-tuning* your body and mind so you can better receive the broadcast that is constantly being sent out by Spirit.

You may find that regular meditation leads you toward life-style changes. For me to tune in, I have had to quit drinking coffee. That doesn't mean I never drink it, but I know that I cannot feel subtle energies when I am jacked on caffeine—or sugar for that matter. Even ingesting a tiny cup of espresso and a cookie interfere with my ability to tune in. Giving up coffee was a slow process. I finally realized I felt so much better without it. I used to live with constant worry. I didn't know the caffeine was causing it.

I recommend that you move toward your meditation position with a sense of commitment, concentration, and comfort. I sit on a pillow. When you sit, keep your spine elongated. The spine is the physical superhighway for the nervous system. A straight spine allows messages to flow from the mind to the body—and the body to the mind. A straight spine acts as an antenna to our higher self. To Spirit.

Note: You can partake in plant medicine ceremonially and reverently before you meditate for deeper and easier access to the subtle energies, but you don't need to. These time-worn meditation practices work on their own. In fact, the medicine can fire and wire the neural pathways for you and then you can practice strengthening those pathways by meditating without medicine. Marijuana is not a short cut to spiritual realization or your spiritual practice. It just helps nudge you in the direction you want to go, by allowing you to feel.

Transcendental Meditation/The Relaxation Response

1. Find a quiet place you will regularly be able to practice in. The Buddha suggested you sit in a forest place under a tree or any other very quiet place.

2. Create a mantra (a word you will repeat over and over that has special meaning to you). Some suggestions are: *One, Love, Peace, Aum, God.* Keep the mantra secret. This is your special word only. Keeping it secret keeps it sacred and more powerful.

3. Set a timer for an allotted amount of time. I suggest you start at 20 minutes. If that feels too long, set the timer for ten minutes. The idea is to find an amount of time you can sit comfortably and practice focusing. Sitting for too long too soon can become uncomfortable—physically and emotionally—and you can end up fighting your own monkey mind. Once you find a time you can comfortably start with, then you can lengthen the time from there, working up to at least 20 minutes and then from there to an hour or more.

4. Sit comfortably cross legged in silence with your spine gently erect. If you feel better in a chair with a straight back, that is perfectly acceptable too. Relax your muscles. Let your body get as soft as it can while your spine stays straight.

5. Say a prayer for help in your quest to feel Spirit. Talk to your higher power about your sincere desire to connect. Pray for forgiveness for any judgments you mistakenly have cast on your brothers and sisters. (Our unconscious judgments of others hold us back. They often are really how we feel about ourselves. We hold our higher Self back when we judge.)

6. Set your intention for your practice—for example, "I intend to concentrate fully in my meditation for the next twenty minutes."

7. Gently close your eyes if you haven't already. Breathe in through the nose. Exhale through the nose, then repeat your mantra, "One." Breathe in, breathe out, repeat mantra "One." Do this over and over. See the breath being inhaled and exhaled—then repeat your sacred mantra.

8. Practice this for the allotted amount of time. If your mind wanders while you practice, gently bring your attention back to your mantra. It becomes easier and easier to concentrate on only your mantra the more you do it. Once your alarm rings, sit in silence for five minutes at least and feel the reverberating effects of your practice.

That's it! It's that simple. Try this every day for a month. As you do, you may notice a growing sense of being cared for and watched over by a benevolent, loving presence.

Hong Sau Meditation

1. Find a quiet place you will be able to regularly practice in.

2. Sit in silence with your spine erect. Relax your muscles while your spine stays lifted. Say a prayer for help in your quest to feel Spirit. Talk to Spirit about your sincere desire to connect. Pray for forgiveness for any judgments you mistakenly have cast on your brothers and sisters.

3. Set a timer for an allotted amount of time. I would start at 20 minutes. If that feels like too much, set it for ten minutes.

4. Close your eyes and gently roll them up so that they are physically rolled towards the center point of your eyebrows—without any strain. Your eyes are focused on the *Ajna* chakra, which is your third eye center. Let the eyes relax while you maintain their slight upward turn.

5. Let the breath slow and elongate. Take even inhales and exhales for a few breaths, then let the breath be. Let the breath come into the lungs on its own accord; when you feel the need to breathe in, do so.

6. On the inhale say silently to yourself, "Hong" rhymes with "song"—and then retain the breath with no

forcing until you feel the need to release it. When you release your breath, silently repeat to yourself "Sau," rhymes with Paw. Do this over and over for twenty minutes or for whatever you've set your timer to. (You may get to a point where you really don't need to immediately inhale and that the space between the breaths becomes longer. And you will find that there are whole worlds that can be accessed in between the breaths.)

7. When your timer rings, relax the inner gaze. Sit silently with the feelings of peace that have been cultivated from the practice.

The Hong Sau technique has an inspiring history behind it. Some observers of Hong Sau chant slightly different words (Ham Sa) which means the same thing— "I am He" or "I am Spirit." Knowing the history and what you are saying when you repeat Hong Sau or any of the other practices I outline can give you an intellectual understanding of the words— but it is by repeating the words and following the directions outlined here that intellectual understanding can bloom into far deeper experience.

Vipassana Meditation

Vipassana meditation is one of the roots of all mindfulness meditation practices and is as old as Siddhartha Gautama, the Buddha. In fact, the Vipassana meditation technique is said to have been discovered by Buddha and is the meditation technique through which the Buddha achieved enlightenment. It is taught in the *Satipatthana Sutta*, Buddha's discourse on mindfulness. It is therefore also the oldest Buddhist meditation technique. However, it can also be practiced by non-Buddhists. Vipassana means "insight" in Sanskrit, and insight into the true nature of reality is the goal of Vipassana. The meditator uses Vipassana meditation to "see things as they are," or to uncover the hidden truth of all existence.

1. Find a quiet place in which you can regularly practice meditation.

2. Sit in silence with your spine lifted. Relax your muscles while your spine stays lifted. Scan your body and make sure there is absolutely no tension in the vehicle (body).

3. Say a prayer for help in your quest to feel Spirit. Talk to Spirit about your sincere desire to connect. Pray for forgiveness for any judgments you mistakenly have cast on your brothers and sisters. (As I have written, our unconscious judgments hold us back; they are really how we feel about ourselves. We hold ourselves back when we judge and we hold our brothers and sisters back when we judge them).

4. Set your intention for your practice (See chapter 7 on Intention.)

5. Set a timer—I would start at 20 minutes. If that feels like too much, try for something shorter like ten minutes.

6. Close your eyes. Start by beginning to focus the attention on your breathing. You start to become aware of your breath only, of the rising and falling of your chest, and how you feel the breath coming out of your nostrils. When this small step is mastered, you can go further with the Vipassana body scan.

7. Next, begin to scan your body in your mind's eye, bit by bit by completely focusing on the sensations of only the specific area you are addressing at the time. You can start at the top of your head.

8. Imagine/experience mentally the top of your head. Begin to scan the top of your head, you can start with the outside of your head. Then, go about an inch inside your skull. Scan from the front top of your forehead towards the back of your head. Experience your hair, hair follicles, the layer of skin, then below that to the bone of your skull and brain underneath that. Now scan across the entire top of your head. I like to see it almost as if I am mowing the lawn—making sure to not leave any part of my head un-scanned.

9. Go slow, take your time. when the entire top first inch of your head is scanned, move the next inch down, here "see" your forehead, skin, skull, part of your brain or frontal lobe, pineal gland, back of the brain or the cerebellum, skin, hair follicles, and hair.

   a. Now, move down another inch and starting from the front again, see your eyelids, lashes, eyebrows, the bridge of your nose, and scan through to the actual cartilage. Keep scanning through to your eyeball and eye socket and behind that.

b. Continue scanning your body in this fashion and go through the entire body. Take your time. Sometimes your attention may wander. Just bring it back to your breath and where you left off on your scan.

c. At the end of the time you have given yourself for meditation, take five minutes to practice Metta. Metta means benevolence, loving-kindness, friendliness, amity, good will, and active interest in others. Silently repeat over and over the following affirmations: "I am filled with loving kindness." Repeat this phrase silently to yourself several times until you feel the words reverberate/emanate through and out of you before you move on to the following phrases. "I am peaceful and at ease," "I am happy and content," and the last one, "I am well."

As you practice any of the above meditations, be aware that as you sit you may have little aches or tics or tiny pains that show up in parts of the body. Try to sit with them as you are, rather than adjusting to get comfortable. This allows you to observe that something has come up. A fidgety body is indicative of a fidgety mind—that means symptoms want to come out. So, sit with whatever comes up.

When we bring this degree of mindfulness to the inner body or to a concentration, we can encounter the "issues in our tissues." One time I was practicing Vipassana meditation and I had a little pain in my leg. I was about to move my leg to a new position when I remembered that I could just watch the pain and not do anything about it. The next thing I knew, I was gently crying as an emotion and painful memory sprang up—seemingly out of nowhere. I felt the feelings, shed some tears and then remembered I was meditating and started right back up where I had left off —somewhere in my stomach area—and continued scanning. The pain in my leg had disappeared.

By the time I was done with the meditation. I felt so free and light, as though a burden had been lifted. Indeed, a burden had lifted. An emotion or feeling I couldn't properly express at the time it happened had lifted up and off my body. I was lighter because I wasn't carrying the heaviness of this emotion in me anymore.

Again, I recommend you practice one of these meditations every day for a month before moving on to another one. The results are subtle. But don't get attached to seeing a result. Just faithfully give yourself the time to meditate every day. I hope that a feeling of lightness—as soft as a butterfly's touch—will come to sit on your shoulder forever.

See if you can keep the feeling of quiet peace with you beyond your meditation time. See if you can use this practice as a bigger practice of observing not only your meditation time but also each moment of your daily and nightly life.

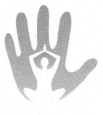

Chapter 10

YOUR BRAIN ON CANNABIS AND YOGA

"So, if we want to change some aspect of our reality, we have to think, feel, and act in new ways; we have to "be" different in terms of our responses to experiences. We have to "become" someone else. We have to create a new state of mind ... we need to observe a new outcome with that new mind." —Joe Dispenza

For some of us, but not all of us, taking part in plant medicine alters our brain in certain ways that allow us to increase our perception of reality. I want to focus on what happens within our body and brain during plant medicine yoga that can create the phenomenon that we might choose to call spiritual experience. I am not a scientist, but I have gathered my information from years of research. I'll explain the energetic and brain chemistry shifts during this practice as I understand them from research and my own experience with plant medicine yoga. Energetically, when you partake in plant medicine you are allowing the plant to amplify what you are concentrating on. When you sit still in meditation before you begin your yoga, your concentration is intensified. Sitting still in concentration tunes your nervous system into a deeper, slower, more balanced vibration. The addition of cannabis adjusts your nervous system so you can more easily experience a deep stillness, a kind of portal through which you might enter into a more expansive plane. The more you practice, the easier it is to drop in. And, I find that the more I practice, the more I get to carry the deeper vibration with me into my daily life as well. The peace that comes with this practice lingers for longer periods of time.

In my research I found that author Joan Bello explains it best. Bello is considered a leading pioneer by many in the medicinal marijuana field. She is the author of *The Benefits of Marijuana, Physical, Psychological and Spiritual*. Her book investigates the process of how cannabis interacts and plays with the body, mind and consciousness. Bello found that marijuana's effects on brain patterns are indirect. She believes the plant's greatest influence is through our Autonomic Nervous System (ANS).

The ANS is a two-branched process made up of the sympathetic and parasympathetic nervous systems. It's a vast communication network of electrochemical signals. Our brain has two processing sides as well, the left and right hemispheres. When THC from cannabis enters the blood stream, its effect on the Autonomic Nervous System is to enhance both sides of the brain. Each side is believed to exert its opposing-complimentary/equalizing influence in a complex neuro-chemical cooperation to balance the body under all conditions. When we interpret our situation as safe, when we are not tired or worried, our autonomic nervous system rests at equilibrium. Because the way we feel reflects and is reflected by our body chemicals, we don't need to ingest any substance from outside our organisms to change our moods when we are relaxed.

But if we have an overwhelm of stress from modern living, such as driving in traffic or being exposed to negative media input or being compulsively busy, we will most likely find ourselves out of balance. The cumulative effect over a number of years of this kind of living wears on our natural ability to maintain balance.

When an over-abundance of sensory and neurological excitement occurs in one moment, the ANS compensates by generating equalizing doses of depressant hormones. This can help us continually balance our energetic responses. But the ANS system can get worn down.

How does marijuana/plant medicine come into play with this natural and complicated balancing act? Cannabis works in the body as a leveler for extreme energy swings. It does not only stimulate. It does not solely depress. Cannabis can facilitate both adjustments simultaneously. Bello calls this cannabis balance in the ANS: "charged equilibrium."

According to Joan Bello, my own experience and the reported experiences of others, many physiological changes occur with marijuana use by most people. Yet none of the changes are extreme in any one direction. The action of marijuana on the body causes slower and more expansive breathing. At the same time, the sacs in the lungs (alveoli) expand so that carbon dioxide is more efficiently eliminated, allowing for greater oxygen intake. When slower and deeper breathing occurs, we are in a highly functioning, yet relaxed system with better fuel. That is why with marijuana use, one can feel both relaxed *and* alert, sometimes experienced as "being high."

How does this internally energized balancing act with cannabis and yoga constitute a spiritual experience? When we reach the state of "charged equilibrium," we know it. We can feel it in our body. Our breath feels slow and even, our body feels balanced—light and fluid. The yoga postures help clear the body of stagnant stuck energies and help balance and quiet the mind. Cannabis amplifies our ability to feel what we are doing and makes us present. When we are in this state, we are receptive to what simply *Is*. We feel free and light and connected to a larger, blissful whole.

We can observe the thoughts and feelings that float in our body without getting triggered by them. There is a neutrality that allows us to observe them as they float through us. This is our natural state. This is the state we were born into as babies, when we were soft and properly breathing with full belly breaths. I believe it may be possible to access this state and space all the time—and live and move from this heightened condition.

What makes Plant Medicine Yoga a spiritual experience or practice? The more we get ourselves into this place of expansion through the yoga and medicine, the easier it is to revisit this same state without the medicine.

Neuropsychologist Donald O. Hebb and more recently Dr. Joe Dispenza say, "neurons that fire together get wired together." This phrase was first used in 1949 to describe how pathways in the brain are formed and reinforced through repetition. The more we perform a certain task, the stronger that neural network in our brain becomes, making the process of whatever we are doing more efficient each successive time. When we practice cannabis yoga, we create neural pathways that lead us to the experience of spiritual connection. This pathway and the ability to access this "high state" is strengthened with repeated practice— with or without the medicine. When you look at the definitions of a spiritual experience, you find *transcendence, merging, feeling connected and whole, bliss, joy, and union.*

I define a spiritual connection as having a peak experience or illumination of some kind that alters our life forever. The proof of the spiritual comes with how we integrate the experience into our life. We can receive amazing insights through the medicine and through our body. But this type of sacred knowledge usually asks us to take an action or make a change in our life of some sort. We alter the way we live. Maybe the action is forgiveness. Maybe we realize we need to let go of a limiting behavior, human connection, or old tired belief. Maybe personal spirituality is as simple as continuing to see something in this broader way.

What separates a spiritual experience from just a great visualization is that the peak experience or epiphany profoundly alters us. Some people experience the spiritual phenomena as a physical healing in their body, while others experience healing in their minds and emotions. And a healing in the mind or emotions can bring about a healing in the body or vice versa. I know the spiritual experience is real when it fosters complete lasting changes with how I interact with myself and the world.

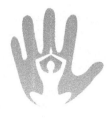

Chapter 11

MAKING LOVE AS A SPIRITUAL OFFERING

"Love is a gift of one's inner most soul to another
so both can be whole." —Buddha

I suppose I've known forever that making love can be a spiritual offering, but to *know* that the possibility exists and to regularly experience spiritual lovemaking are different— profoundly different. The power of Santa Maria, combined with aware movement, can carry beyond the length of a yoga class into every moment of your life, *including* your love life.

When I first started teaching Sacred Plant Medicine, I had already experienced what felt like an intense charge of electricity circulating throughout my body. It was an energy current that continually washed through my entire body from the crown of my head to my toes. And from my toes up through my crown. This powerful flow stayed with me after every weekly yoga class.

You might assume that the raised flow of energy and the higher charge coursing through my body would have created more fuel for passion between my husband and me in our lovemaking. After all, Sacred Plant Medicine Yoga was infusing passion in every other area of my life. But that wasn't the case for our sexual connection, our passion connection. The heightened flow coming through me didn't make our love more intense. It did the opposite...at first.

In my early teaching days, when I first came home from a class, I was highly sensitive to everything. I'd walk in the door and feel blasted by fluorescent glare from the kitchen light—on my skin and in my eyes. I had to go straight outside where I resumed doing yoga or sat in meditation watching the sun drop below the horizon.

I got the space I needed when I went outside, space that absorbed the extra high voltage energy I felt. I didn't know about grounding the yogic raised energy in the beginning of my teaching cannabis yoga. What came through during class was far more powerful than what could be contained in a living room or inside any dwelling. I learned that I needed nature without human influence or presence after a class. Sometimes I walked our dog Yogi in companionable silence. When I began going outside after teaching, Brent volunteered to accompany me. And although I loved sharing walks with him, I needed time to let the energy from class drain and slow its course. Conversation brought more energies in. I needed to do nothing else but bring silent mindfulness to my walking. I tried to explain what I needed to my husband. "Angel, yes of course come, but I can't talk. I just need to breathe." What I didn't know at the time, but have since come to understand, is I was learning how to balance and ground the amplified energy in my nervous system. Having Brent's energy in my presence right after a class didn't allow for the release and return to ground that I needed.

Initially he didn't understand my need to be alone. We had always shared our walks and would talk and solve the world's problems big and small while we covered walking trails and wild land. But under the influence, I could no longer do the kind of walking and talking that required me to jump back into my analytical mind. I was humming with more life force then I could easily experience. I needed to *feel*, stay out of the thinking mind and connect with the earth beneath me. I needed to just BE.

My new way of "being" started to drive a wedge between Brent and me. This need to *be* was the need to be present. Nothing else had changed between us except I was feeling everything more, which means I was increasingly more present to what was in front of me. Brent was still the loving man he always had been. But I had changed. What was coursing through me created changes in the level of presence I was bringing to almost everything.

Suddenly, there was a misconnect in our marriage. We were no longer on the same wavelength. If he came to yoga class with me—the growing chasm between us could shorten. When Brent attended class, he also experienced the cleansing release and new flow of vitality that we all did. After class, he felt the same need to ground. The life-changing effects of the class lingered for the rest of the night for both of us. But for him, it would fade by the next morning. For me the effects remained.

If he didn't attend my class, we couldn't connect at all when I came home because we were in two different vibrations. This disconnect started to affect our daily life which, of course, carried over into our love life. We slowly began to find ourselves incapable of deeply connecting.

I took time to go into myself. My sexual self. It dawned on me that to make love in the past, I had always compartmentalized. I played whatever role I knew my lover needed, just as in daily life, I often played the role of wife, mother, friend, career person. I would sense the other's need or expectation and become what he needed. In order to be the desirable chameleon, I felt I had to box up the rest of me and take on the color of what each situation was asking for.

But, as I became more and more authentic in my practice, I could no longer shape-shift, especially when I was making love. I wanted to make love with my whole being, not a relegated, and somewhat artificial fragment of myself. Brent didn't know what was going on. He felt frustrated and rejected and I didn't know what was going on or how to explain what I was experiencing.

My newfound sensitivities allowed me to experience states of bliss in my class and meditation that brought me higher than I had ever experienced. But when it came time to share that bliss through my body with him, I shut down. If Brent wasn't ultra-sensitive, as I was, I couldn't be intimate with him.

The online dictionary defines ultra as: very; extremely. Sensitive is defined as: having or displaying a quick and delicate appreciation of others' feelings. What I needed so that we could meet and connect within my expansive awareness was my husband's full-on appreciation of my new-found feelings.

I needed to feel love—from me to Brent, from him to me. I needed not lust, not power, not stress relief, not anything but my partner's full love, appreciation, sensitivity, and attention—without the ruling goal of orgasm. I usually just flow in all matters. But I could not just flow with this newfound energy expressing itself through me.

The deepest part of me knew that, to be truly connected to myself and another person physically and sexually, I needed to let go and be present. Present with what is, present in this moment. Before, in the past, whenever it came to love-making, I would get myself a "pre-love" drink—some kind of alcohol, a beer, or a glass of wine. Then I could soften and get a little numb and perform according to whatever my lover was asking for—or I was asking myself to do. In the past, alcohol would help me relax, it would blur boundaries and help me move from one activity, perhaps dinner with friends, the drive home and into the bedroom for intimacy—whether I felt connected to my husband or not. After I started practicing Sacred Plant Medicine Yoga and became more connected to all of me, I could no longer just have sex.

After just weeks of practicing Sacred Plant Medicine Yoga, I began to see the sacred in the every-day, including and especially in my body, my un-altered body. I had spent my life forcing my body to look a certain way, act a certain way and be what I thought others expected and wanted. Through plant medicine yoga, I was done forcing anything on myself.

And I stopped taking that glass of wine to relax. That glass of wine, I realized, wasn't just to relax. It was a muzzle I put on the little girl inside of me, so I could carry on according to my "will." In essence I was drugging her into submission, so she would shut up.

Now, with this new appreciation of me and my spirit, I took the glass of wine only when I wanted wine and I found I wanted it less and less. I let myself feel exactly whatever I was feeling and honored the knowing by acting accordingly. If I was going to stay present to the higher energies that were now running my body, mind, and spirit, I needed to honor my body in all my affairs. It was time to listen to and honor the subtle finer, higher energies that move and permeate within and around the body vessel and all it is. Once I found this connection to "all of me," I determined to never lose touch with this delicate, ephemeral me ever again. This meant above all else, I needed to honor my feelings.

If we went straight to my private parts the minute we lay down, I didn't feel loved. I didn't feel cherished. And the truth of the matter was my whole me wasn't being loved and I wasn't being cherished. I realized what I needed when we made love was the same connected let-go-of-everything-else-except-this-moment kind of consciousness that I had learned to give myself in my hour and a half yoga class.

Making love with my lover was not really different, since it involved the mixing and union of not only one body, mind, and spirit, but *two* connected bodies, minds and spirits. I needed and wanted totally present love—and if love expressed itself through the body in sexual touch, then great. If it expressed itself through the body in loving gazes that allowed us to get in touch with the highest and best in each other, then great. But I could no longer just "do sex." I could only make aware and present love with my aware and present body.

I didn't know how to say any of this to my beloved husband. I didn't have the words to articulate what I was experiencing. I didn't know who it was that suddenly had these needs and wanted to express them this way. I found making love was exactly like my yoga, I had to be present in my body and I needed to bring the same mindfulness to my union with Brent. I needed to let go of everything I was doing up until that point and let go of everything I was going to be doing after *and* everything I thought he wanted or I thought I should be doing, and I needed to give myself permission to be present, with one hundred percent mindfulness.

Aware and present love translated into physically lying with him, feeling him, touching his skin, and administering love and attention to his body, mind, and spirit—and to *my* body, mind, and spirit. I was no longer going to—and wasn't able even if I wanted to—"will" myself to be what I thought and imagined anyone needed of me.

If someone wanted me to be a certain way so they could be happy and it didn't vibe with my own highest expression at the time, my time of being a chameleon was no longer possible. This was a huge departure from the "people pleasing" person I'd been my entire life. This higher vibration I was living in could not be compartmentalized to fit any kind of box, container, or definition of how I should be. Especially how I made love.

What was new for me when I was making love was staying tuned into my body and keeping my body soft while my energy was mixing with my husband's. If I was completely present, I was all the way there, feeling what was going on within me physically, emotionally, and mentally—and I was feeling *him* in the same way. I had never made love that way before. Making love is literally loving on each other and ourselves. It's totally different from sex. And, making present and aware love was scary for me.

In my lifetime, I have experienced some of the many different ways we can "make love" and "have sex." I experienced the passion that comes with discovering a new love and the ache from being separated from that love. I've experienced the fierce love that comes when we reunite with our beloved. I've also experienced sex in its different guises: drunken sex and quickies, make-up sex and miss you sex and "I'm not in the mood sex" and dress up and play a role sex, beautiful dinner followed by sex and "I owe you something sex," sex outdoors, sex on the beach, sex in the pouring rain. But I had only rarely experienced mystically (as in a divine gift or blessing) lovemaking as full-on union with another in body, mind, and spirit. I had only rarely experienced transcendent love that brought me to tears and brought me to new realms and brought me to spiritual unification through another.

"Conscious" lovemaking was brand new territory for me. It made me feel extremely vulnerable because I could no longer hide behind a role. It felt like I had accessed the purity in me and once I felt that divine female light in my core, I knew I could never compromise her to make someone else feel comfortable, unless it made me feel comfortable as well.

My husband and I arrived at a crossroad. We almost didn't know how to navigate. We still loved each other, but neither one of us was getting the physical love and touch we needed from the other. Brent and I talked about my reluctance to "have sex." I volunteered to go to a marriage counselor or a sex therapist. I looked into identical hormones which address changing hormones in the body that can affect sexual desire and I even got an "O" shot, a series of shots that injects your own blood platelets into your genitals so you are re-energized.

Brent and I wondered if the problem was lack of desire. But that was never the problem. The problem was we were coming from two different vibrations. This mis-connect continued on and off for about a year and we both felt more estranged daily.

Then, Brent did something he had been talking about for years. And that made all the difference. He started meditating. He had been saying for years that he wanted to join me in meditation, and he would try either with me or on his own. But sitting was difficult. He ended up fighting with himself. He couldn't let go of the thoughts that churned in his mind. He couldn't be quiet. Something as simple as just sitting in silence was torturous. He tried. But he could never contain or channel his high energy long enough to sit still or focus on one thing for a period of time.

I had the same problem when I used to drink coffee. Once I quit caffeine it got easier. But Brent was already off stimulants. He has always had high energy. It worked well in the world because he could get things done. The world considered him very successful. But his energy had gotten out of balance, as mine had.

In February of 2019, Brent was invited into a ten-day silent meditation course at a place called Quepasana in Maui, Hawaii. There, he learned a meditation style that gave him a way to slow his racing thoughts and calm his mind. It involved more than just sitting with a mantra; he learned Vipassana meditation.

When the course was over. Brent continued practicing this new-found meditation every morning. As his practice continued, we both noticed outward signs of an inner transformation. He became more peaceful. Instead of talking all the time, he listened more. He slowed his walk and instead of running from one activity to the next, he completed what he was doing and then moved slowly with ease and even grace to the next. Instead of constantly being on the phone while we were driving, he just drove. He took the time to notice the landscape, the cars, the drivers—and he took the time to notice me. We both saw the signs of his deepening connection to an invisible peace—that union rippled through him to me, flowed into our lovemaking and into something so grand, so high, and so big that through it we were catapulted into new worlds together.

It started with both of us becoming aware of our senses. Sometimes we would partake in cannabis beforehand, sometimes we didn't. We were already at the same vibration of being present with each other. It started with the environment we created before we lay down to be close. For me it started with an intention for union and connection, feeling my feelings and feeling his. Brent and I were able to create deep connection with each other when we stopped everything else and brought awareness to our senses and deep inner feelings.

Just as we might do in the Sacred Plant Medicine Yoga class, we suspend discussion, slow down, take full, slow, even belly-breaths. This all helps us get present and relaxed. Once we are relaxed, we tune in to our five senses. We become aware of what we are seeing, hearing, tasting, smelling, and feeling. (The bed and comforter under me, his hands on my arms, the beauty of the candlelight, the smell of orange blossoms from the candle.)

We both now realize that any time we are focused on the moment, we are practicing meditation. We light candles throughout the bedroom and turn on music that allows us to open our hearts and create a connected flow. We lie together and hold each other. We breathe together, massage each other. We use our senses to connect, which brings us to a space we can only access through our bodies.

We are past thinking. We came here through feeling. We came here through the senses. We have made love with candles and music many times before, but what makes this intimacy different is there is no goal to do or be anything other than to share and connect in deep sacred intimacy and sensuality. I came to understand I have been afraid of being this close to another person.

BREATHE

The cannabis combined with mindfulness from our meditation and yoga has led us again to an ancient practice. We have stumbled onto tantric yoga, a practice that promotes sexual spirituality and emotional interconnectedness. Tantra honors and celebrates our bodies, and enriches sensual pleasure, not just sexual pleasure. We acknowledge breath, meditation, mindfulness, movement, eye gazing, and our environment to enhance intimacy with ourselves and each other. The mindfulness we cultivate from our practices of meditation and Sacred Plant Medicine Yoga have carried over, for both of us, to an awareness of how to occupy the body as a way to transcend the physical—and merge into each other's energy and the cosmos.

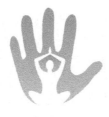

Chapter 12

A FEMININE REVOLUTION WILL SAVE THE EARTH

"How is it possible that the most intellectual creature to ever walk the planet Earth is destroying its only home?" —Jane Goodall

If you would have told me five years ago that plants house an intelligent spirit that can communicate with us, I would honestly have thought you were crazy. I would have thought you were delusional, maybe nice...perhaps, but slightly off. I would have listened to you in interest, but my deepest thought would be, "It's not possible." And I would have dismissed the conversation as not being relevant. And I would have gone on in my rushed life, drinking my coffee and reaching for my sugar throughout the day and having my wine with dinner, even though I didn't really always enjoy the effects. And I would have continued buying my outfits from time to time, to stay current with the fashions, and I would have continued celebrating my Christmases with my family, but wishing desperately that the spirit of it would come back. In other words, I would have moved on past our conversation, filed it away as nonsense and continued to function in the world, all the while knowing that some deep intrinsic element was missing. I would have kept sleep-running (not walking) through my life, donning the various roles society placed on me, until I died.

But I tried plant medicine. I was open enough to say, "What *is* it that our forefathers and mothers were doing when they went on vision quests, what *is* it that some people experience when they do cannabis or ayahuasca, mushrooms or peyote? And why did early man or indigenous people from all around the world form all these various rituals around plants?

And I got my answer. Like millions before me, I experienced, first-hand, deep, physical, spiritual, and emotional healing. I gained insights into family patterns, I released generations of family shame I didn't know I was carrying in my body. I realized along with the physical traits we inherit from our family—like our eye color—we also inherit our family's emotional and psychological traits. My various plant medicine journeys helped me forgive those who hurt me. And I forgave myself for the pain I inadvertently caused others. When I went on journeys and did my own deep healing sacred plant medicine yoga, I was physically once-and-for-all relieved of aches and pains that had plagued me for years. The work freed me, and I felt clean.

But I didn't leave those yoga and introspective journey sessions and just continue on my merry way—picking up where I left off. The experiences left such a deep impression that, in order to be in full integrity with myself, I had to integrate their teachings in my everyday life.

The plant medicine yoga helped me see that **what had been missing from my life—most of my life—was me.** The wild, alive, passionate, free, lover of all of life me. She had been boxed in, cornered, subjugated, conformed, enslaved, brow-beaten into submission and what was left of her was an anxious, neurotic people-pleaser, who was good at playing whatever role you most needed filled at the moment. I was a contracted, shallow breathing, constantly apologizing woman who had learned to dress to please, who had learned to say the right words to please, who had learned to please period.

The medicine made it very apparent that what had disappeared from my life and what I see missing in so many of our lives is the actual *life force energy which animates and gives us life.* Life force energy is another name for spirit. I needed spirit. I needed more of the stuff that animates. What I now know, but didn't know then, is life force is physically brought in through the breath. I needed prana. Prana is defined in the dictionary as: breath. It is not only breath we need. It is *all* that rides on oxygen's invisible current. And we need more of it. Most of us are dying for real life force. We need more vitality. I'm not talking about the fake, nervous, anxiety-producing energy that comes from stimulants like caffeine and sugar. We need the lightness of spirit that comes from drinking in fresh oxygenated air from outside. The lightness of spirit that comes from eating vital nutrient-rich vegetables and fruits. We need this so we can *feel* our life.

I believe that there is a quiet revolution rallying inside many of us. And I believe it is a feminine revolution. It is a call to both men and women alike to embrace all things that protect and preserve nature. How does that invisible call appear in my life? How do I make my answer visible? Tangible? I continually make concrete changes in how I am living. I take new actions that align with the truth that we only have a few short years left to turn around the trajectory of where our planet is headed, before it's too late. (And, there are more than a few wise people suggesting that it is already too late. That is no excuse to continue using the earth as an infinite source).

What is a feminine revolution? It is a return to feeling ourselves. It is a return to respecting our own voice and lovingly speaking our truth. This feminine revolution is not gender specific. I am not just talking about women in a feminine revolution. I am talking about all humans honoring the feminine in each of ourselves. That means, as a society, as a group of people, we need to value and respect and practice feminine traits like connection, empathy, nurturing, feeling, emoting, listening and receiving. In short, LOVING has to be central to all we do.

To embrace my feminine self, I needed to let myself feel my real power, my real glory, my real voice and I needed to live unapologetically with who I was from here on out.

As I practiced lovingly listening and speaking my truth, as I started to wear what felt good versus what was in fashion, as I started eating and drinking according to how I felt, the tiny flickering of a flame inside me grew steadier. This individual healing that can spring from cannabis yoga can't help but effect the whole. Me living my truth will have an influence on those around me, my family, my friends— just because I am in proximity with them.

By embracing myself, I became more aware of my connection with Mother Earth. We need to get back out in nature and re-member (as in become a member again) our connection with her. We need to feel the heartbeat of our mother by walking barefoot on her land. We need to sit in the sun and absorb its healing light into our bodies. We need to swim in her oceans and wade in her streams. We need to climb her mountains and we need to love and enjoy her. Nature holds the source of our prana. En masse, we are not getting enough of it. Our lifestyles have slowly cut us off from our source. What we feel is real. Our feelings are more real than everything else. How we feel when we hold something in our hands and how we feel when someone says a biting remark define our reality. What we feel puts us in touch with where we are. It is the single most spectacular gift of being alive. It brings us to the present moment. And that is the place where we have power to make true conscious choices. We can pause all the time to just do nothing but feel.

The Greek philosopher Socrates said, "The unexamined life is not worth living." What he was saying is, if we do not pause and look at what we are doing, at the choices we are making, chances are we are running on auto pilot. Which means we—the *we* that is supposedly steering our ship and making the choices in our life—is no longer in there. We've reduced ourselves to being a combination of societal programs. When that happens, we are no longer vitally, creatively alive, which leads us as a society, to quote Henry David Thoreau, to just men (and women) leading lives of quiet desperation. This fragmenting of the self creates the breeding ground for becoming ruled by habits and addictions (as does trauma and pain of all kinds).

When we feel, we get to live our lives without projections and judgments and get to see it and be there as it is unfolding. That means we are truly alive. When we are this awake, we are connected to ourselves, each other and Mother Earth. When we are connected with ourselves, then we know what it is we need to do now or in the next moment. We know what we came here to do. We are in touch with our purpose. We know because we can *feel* it. Our internal guidance system is always pointing us to our truth north. We can feel when we are on course and pointed in the right direction. Plant medicine can help us more easily see that.

For some of us, feeling so much can be scary. Feeling our feelings can be so exquisitely painful that we almost can't bear it. I'm including even good or positive feelings. Many of us have learned coping mechanisms to help us maneuver through our days so we don't have to feel so much. In the process of avoiding feelings, we develop habits that keep us locked in little cocoons or bubbles. What happens as we block negative feelings, though, is we also block positive feelings like joy and peace and we forget that we are intrinsically connected to each other and the earth. When we lose the feeling of connectedness, we start believing we are alone.

Plant medicines can help you remember who you are.

If you've read this far, maybe that means you are open to the idea that plants actually have the power to connect us to our deepest self and connect us to the breath of life, to all that is. There are other things out there that can help us wake up. Almost any experience can be a call to awaken. The most direct path for me has been through cannabis and other entheogenic plants. As we learned in the "History of Cannabis" chapter, visionary plants have been used by indigenous people for thousands of years. People are returning to the plant medicines of ancient ancestors and its practices in huge numbers because as a species we are searching for meaning and connection and healing in our lives.

A U.S. population survey found there were approximately 32 million lifetime psychedelic users in 2010. Those numbers are growing. As we awaken to all that psychoactive plants offer, we are also being called by them to take responsibility for our lives. The plants are helping us reconnect to the parts of ourselves that *know* we are connected to each other and the earth. The plants are helping us re-member and re-join with each other under one earth nation, so that we can save our home and ourselves. This may sound like a science fiction movie but look at the science. We are destroying ourselves and we are reaching an irreversible tipping point. We have only a few years to turn the trajectory of our planet around or we will kill her, which means we destroy ourselves.

Individually, cannabis and other psychoactive substances can help us heal from experiences, and integrate and release trauma from our body. But that is just the first step in the healing work offered by these plants. Clearing the traumas from our body puts us in touch with who we really are at the core of our being, and that is light. We clear the darkness or dross out of our physical and energetic bodies with each journey we take. Dross can build up over a lifetime and it can cover our connection to our own source, or our own light. Picture sludge and dark cellophane that covers up the body or gets trapped in joints. If enough of this accumulates over a lifetime, we can become inflamed and can contract other diseases. Energetically we are slowly blocked from our own light. It's just like when a cloud blocks us from the sun. We see its outline through the cloud, but we no longer feel its life-giving energy. When this happens, we start to see the sun as an abstract object. We lose awareness that it is the giver of *ALL* life on this planet. When that happens, we become caught up in the old system of programming that has been handed down to us from society.

Once we try plant medicines or something like them that help us awaken, we have the opportunity to not only heal our body and mind and reconnect with our true essence, but we realize our connection with each other and the Earth.

And this is where I feel the deeper message from the plants is revealed. As many of us begin to wake up, we are realizing that we have let our living planet spin dangerously toward the extinction of all precious life, including our own. We have gotten so caught up in material things and in illusions and projections, that we have lost the fact that our desire for continuously more and more things are stripping the earth of its precious resources that keep it and us alive. We are out of balance and the plants are helping us see this truth. The more sensitive you are, the more you realize this as well. Scientists are telling us, environmentalists are telling us, economists are telling us, the state of our government is telling us. We have started spinning out of control and we need to take drastic and radical action. The plants are telling me we need to turn back to our roots to regain our balance. What does that look like? When I tune in to the wisdom of *my* body, what I feel in my bones... is we need to become stewards of the earth again.

What is a steward of the earth? Being a steward of the earth is best described, for me, by Chief Luther Standing Bear, who said this about the Lakota tribe: "*The Lakota was a true naturist — a lover of nature. The old people came literally to love the soil, and they sat or reclined on the ground with a feeling of being close to a mothering power. It was good for the skin to touch the earth, and the old people liked to remove their moccasins and walk with bare feet on the sacred earth. Their tipis were built upon the earth and their altars were made of earth. The birds that flew in the air came to rest upon the earth, and it was the final abiding place of all things that lived and grew. The soul was soothing, strengthening, cleansing, and healing. This is why the old Indian still sits upon the earth instead of propping himself up and away from its life-giving forces. For him, to sit or lie upon the ground is to be able to think more deeply and to feel more keenly. He can see more clearly into the mysteries of life and come closer in kinship to other lives about him...The old Lakota was wise. He knew that man's heart away from nature becomes hard; he knew that lack of respect for growing, living things soon led to lack of respect for humans too. So, he kept his youth close to its softening influence."*

I am being called to take active measures to protect our oceans, to eat vegetarian or vegan, to protect our lands and our animals and the shrinking ozone layer, and to live in cooperation with all nations. As a day-to-day practice, that means cooperating with my brothers and sisters. It means *seeing* each stranger as my brother and sister. For me, it means going so slow that I can feel my body all the time and that I consciously breathe all the time. When I take Santa Maria into my body, I clearly see we cannot continue living in the world the way our parents did. We need to work with nature, not control it. We need to understand the preciousness of every life and do what we can to protect and honor it.

It may seem that my suggestions are too radical to actually integrate into your life, but when you look at what I am suggesting, you might find tiny actions you can take that can make a difference and help save our planet. Please refer to the list in the appendix of this book for more steps you can take that will make a difference starting now!

Chapter 13

THE FUTURE—WHERE DO WE GO FROM HERE?

Today, after several decades of suppression and neglect, psychedelics are having a renaissance. A new generation of scientists, many of them inspired by their own personal experience of the compounds, are testing their potential to heal mental illnesses such as depression, anxiety, trauma, and addiction. Other scientists are using psychedelics in conjunction with new brain-imaging tools to explore the links between brain and mind, hoping to unravel some of the mysteries of consciousness. —Michael Pollan (Author of How To Change Your Mind)

I sit cross-legged on a thin mattress. Fifty other people are with me in a big darkened room. We each prepare for what comes next, straighten our mats, adjust our loose clothing, slow our breaths. The woman nearest me clutches a big teddy bear. I brought my trusty Mala beads. She and I—and the others in this room are preparing for deep work. I don't know what might come up for me and I am apprehensive. I do know that we are about to explore the possibilities of utilizing psychedelic plants in a new way—and I am in respectful and uneasy awe.

A deep worshipful repetitively chanted "om" begins to play on the sound system. The ceremony begins. We give thanks to the *Cannabis Sativa* plant for all that it offers before we inhale Her smoke in as sacrament. We recognize and honor the seven directions and what they signify. As each direction is spoken, each participant can take a draw of cannabis smoke from his or her pipe. I inhale only twice.

I'm starting conservatively because I've heard taking Santa Maria in this "psychedelic" way can be powerful. I lie back and let my body relax. The reverential "om" shifts into swirling sounds of crystal bowls and synthesizers. I feel circular vibrations revolving through me all at once. The music swells and expands through me—along with my blood and breath. I follow the music deep inside myself, deep inside my mind and my heart.

The melodies slowly change to sounds of outer space. Random thoughts, almost as if freed from gravity, begin to glide up and drift past me. I look at them and see them for what they are: isolated thought forms attached to nothing. I feel the familiar and welcome sense of light and spaciousness I've come to know from doing cannabis and yoga—but with this more powerful blend of psychedelic cannabis and sound, I experience and feel visions. The music and medicine transport me and my body into the spaciousness of the cosmos.

I drift among planets, stars...and thoughts that look like chemical symbols. More visions come. Past experiences emerge. Some memories bring me to tears, some to deep realizations, some give me insight into my loved ones and my body's health. These different visions all ultimately allow me to see, and more importantly *feel,* past my usual limited understanding.

I sense that hours have gone by, but I've lost all track of time. Our journey is winding down. Our guide, Daniel McQueen, coaxes us slowly back into three-dimensional time with a loving soft voice. "Breathing, breathing, breathing," he says. "Gently bring your awareness back into the room, into the felt experience of your mattress."

I find my mala beads where I have dropped them on the mat, and press them between my fingers, grounding myself with their familiar touch. I reach for my notebook and pen and begin searching for words to describe what I learned and saw. This is my first *guided* psychedelic cannabis experience and It was as deep as my first lone experience with cannabis sativa up in the loft in that Colorado home. And it was as strong and deep as my visits with psilocybin (the active ingredient in magic mushrooms) or even ayuhuasca.

Here. Now. My expectations of cannabis as a psychedelic are confirmed. And experiencing the sacred plant being facilitated in this way with a large group fills me with wonder and hope for what this could mean for transformational healing for the planet...through increased awareness in Her human inhabitants.

A scene which might have appeared to be nothing more than people lying on mats listening to music—like a "nap time for grownups"—is really nothing less than whole body, mind, and spirit medicine work in the highest degree. It is spiritual triage.

We are battle-weary folks lying here and we have each come for different purposes. We have urgencies and needs that go far deeper than the care of just our physical bodies. Here, in this sacred space, we are receiving spiritual medicine through psychedelic cannabis and sound healing. Each of us is a spiritual warrior, each of us is hemorrhaging in ways and from wounds invisible to the human eye.

But this place and these guides—human and plant— offer refuge, deep compassion, space to feel and heal. We have been given profound abiding safety to explore and touch the innate healer that lies within them.

Daniel McQueen, our human guide, is a visionary, and the founder of an international group called Medicinal Mindfulness. He is a Transpersonal Psychedelic Therapist as well as the author of the book, *Psychedelic Cannabis, Breaking the Gate*. McQueen and his group offer regular transformative gatherings in the form of teaching retreats, one-on-one sessions and group gatherings he calls, "Conscious Cannabis Circles."

McQueen has evolved a way to work with cannabis which potentiates its therapeutic and psychoactive properties to elicit deep, safe, and healing psychedelic states.

Since the inception of Medicinal Mindfulness in 2012, he's worked with thousands of people and the results have been staggeringly positive. Many participants have shared stories of personal transformation after working with him.

The numbers of people using psychedelics is rising. According to a July 2020 article in *Scientific American,* called *Americans Increase LSD Use—And A Bleak Outlook for the World May Be to Blame,* by Rachel Nuwar, the number of people using LSD (the psychedelic studied in that report) from 2015 to 2018, increased by more than 50 percent in the U.S.— The authors of the study suspect that many users may be self-medicating to find relief from depression, anxiety, and general stress over the state of the world. The rise was especially pronounced in certain user groups, including people with college degrees (who saw a 70 percent increase) and people aged 26 to 34 (59 percent), 35 to 49 (223 percent), and 50 or older (45 percent). Younger people aged 18 to 25, on the other hand, decreased their use by 24 percent. Andrew Yockey, a doctoral candidate in health education at the University of Cincinnati and lead author of the paper says: "LSD is used primarily to escape. And given that the world's on fire, people might be using it as a therapeutic mechanism." He adds, "Now that COVID's hit, I'd guess that use has probably tripled."

More people are seeking psychedelic alternative healing methods, because increasing numbers of us are suffering from PTSD, trauma, anxieties and addiction. I believe everyone who is living today experiences anxiety. And conventional methods to deal with the rising numbers of us aren't working. According to the US Department of Veterans Affairs, about 6 of every 10 men (or 60%) and 5 of every 10 women (or 50%) experience at least one trauma in their lives. The VA states that: Women are more likely to experience sexual assault and child sexual abuse. Men are more likely to experience accidents, physical assault, combat, disaster, or to witness death or injury. Talk therapy and anti-depressants can't fully penetrate the core of these wounds. But psychedelics can. They have been proven in governmental clinical trials to help heal psychological and emotional injuries where traditional therapies have failed.

Another *Scientific American* article entitled, John Hopkins Scientists Give *Psychedelics the Serious Treatment*, by Tanya Lewis, published in January 2020, discusses how Johns Hopkins Center for Psychedelic and Consciousness Research is exploring the use of psychedelics—primarily psilocybin—for problems ranging from smoking addiction to anorexia and Alzheimer's disease. "One of the remarkably interesting features of working with psychedelics is they're likely to have trans-diagnostic applicability," says Roland R. Griffiths, PhD. In other words, there are multiple benefits for different co-existing symptoms.

Griffiths heads the Johns Hopkins' Center for Psychedelic and Consciousness Research and has led some of the most promising studies evaluating psilocybin for treating depression and alcoholism. His research is backed by MAPS, the Multidisciplinary Association of Psychedelic Studies (MAPS has been leading the way in psychedelic studies since its beginning in 1986).

Griffiths and his colleagues published a foundational study in 2006 showing that a single dose of psilocybin was safe and could cause sustained positive effects and even "mystical experiences." Ten years later they published a randomized double-blind study showing psilocybin significantly decreased depression and anxiety in patients with life-threatening cancer. Each participant underwent two sessions (a high-dose one and a low-dose one) five weeks apart. Six months afterward, about 80 percent of the patients were still less clinically depressed and anxious than before the treatment. Some even said they had lost their fear of death.

Despite findings like these, the major (classically recognized) psychedelics like LSD, psilocybin, Ibogaine, ayuhuasca and MDMA aren't legal yet. People can be thrown in jail for using them for their PTSD, trauma and anxiety—as can "underground" therapists who risk their very freedom by offering this kind of healing work. That means millions of people still continue to suffer every day with life-time traumas they carry and shouldn't have to.

Cannabis is legal and available in many states right now, with more states expected to follow. In the states where cannabis is legal, people can experience cannabis-assisted psychedelic healing right now and stay within the law. Cannabis *Is* a psychedelic. McQueen points out in his book that, "Cannabis is the first psychedelic to break free from the confines of not just the law in some places, but even the clinical and medical models that limit and regulate psychedelic medicine use." Cannabis is paving the way for other psychedelic medicines.

McQueen's message is critical and urgent: "...We need healing and transformation now on the largest scale possible so we can successfully navigate the daily struggles of a world in constant and ever-accelerating global paradigm shifts. In an age where collective trauma is rampant (and seems to only be getting worse), we need to re-evaluate and assess all of the options available to us. *Cannabis sativa*, although previously overlooked, might be one of our best tools to implement psychedelic therapy on a large scale."

Our current laws sanction and even approve various poisons, including alcohol and cigarettes. These are drugs that destroy lives and feed addictions. And yet one of the most striking things about the recent psychedelic research is that the medicines do not appear to be addictive or have adverse effects **when a guide is involved**. Many researchers believe these drugs, which includes cannabis, when used under the supervision of trained professionals, could revolutionize mental health care. Based on my own experience, hundreds of conversations, and my research, I've come to believe cannabis-assisted psychedelics and psychedelics in general are the "healing of the future." And the future is now.

A practical benefit to working with cannabis as a psychedelic, as opposed to others, is that cannabis psychedelic experiences are oftentimes easier to integrate into your everyday waking life. If you've had powerful epiphanies, it's easier to go on to take what you learned and live differently and make new choices—as you see things from a broader perspective. McQueen says using cannabis-assisted psychedelics, "increases the potential for post-session integration." Meaning, you can more easily apply what you learned because you have better access to your newfound insights. After working with Santa Maria in my own way, I believe the plant's greatest gift is in its ability to help us heal and weave that healing into deep personal evolvement.

What does the future look like for Cannabis when the plant is used as an emotional and spiritual healing tool in the ways described in this book? How might our interaction with the plant evolve in the future? How else might this plant ally aid our human family towards further spiritual evolution and awakening? Where could the mindful use of cannabis take us? I believe I stumbled upon answers to these questions when I discovered Medicinal Mindfulness.

The human race stands at a precipice of awakening, and each choice we make and action we take has deep reverberating effects. Our choices now will cast every single one of us, on this planet, into a specific future. Once we are there, we will be stuck with the consequences of our decisions. There will be no way to back out of this future.

If there is a plant that makes us more aware of whether our thoughts and actions serve us, humankind and our delicately balanced and besieged planet, why wouldn't we rush to make great use of that plant's healing gifts?

In continuing to look for answers to these questions, my practice of yoga and cannabis has taken me here in 2020, where I am now enrolled in Medicinal Mindfulness Training. I am learning and practicing the skills of facilitating Cannabis-Assisted Psychedelic therapy for people in need through my Sacred Plant Medicine Journeys based out of Maui, Hawaii. I believe that there is no end to the healing gifts we receive from Santa Maria. And, I am grateful. *Thank you, Santa Maria.*

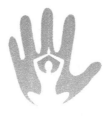

Chapter 14

A GENTLE CAUTION

We all wish for world peace, but world peace will never be achieved unless we first establish peace within our own minds." —Geshe Kelsang Gyatso

May I caution you before you undertake any of the prescribed actions detailed here in this book? Please be careful. Please be mindful. Please use your discernment. Please listen to yourself.

To invoke *Santa Maria* in a spiritual practice calls in the medicinal healing spirit of the plant—in many ways: physically, emotionally, spiritually, psychologically. If you have never interacted with the plant before as a spiritual sacrament or with spiritual intention, you may be startled by the practice's power, the direction, the guidance. I'd like to share some guidelines from my own experience and knowledge before—and as you start to develop your own practice. I want to make sure anyone reading this book understands that working with cannabis in the way it's prescribed here, as an *entheogen*, is like working with something as powerful and as volatile as fire.

Cannabis may not be for everyone. Please know that you may be opening a door that potentially can give you access to every part of you—even the denied parts of you that you have not wanted to see—the dark, sabotaging, hurtful parts of you, and, perhaps more crucially, the denied brilliance, greatness or light inside of you.

Marijuana is an extraordinarily powerful plant medicine. To take it lightly is to misuse its ability to offer deep transformational healing. In my experience, working with the plant as a spiritual ally is similar to taking part in ten years of therapy in one night. If you are not prepared for the journey into yourself, into your psyche, it can be overwhelming—and/or alarming.

Doing sacred plant medicine yoga can expose us to our shadows, those parts of our personality we've held back and pushed down. This practice can also illuminate repressed memories. Working with the plant helps bring long-buried traumas to the surface, so we can feel them and heal them. When we are psychologically ready, becoming aware of and feeling our shadows can be very freeing. Especially when we can integrate what we learn into our life and live more wholly, more holy.

As can fire, plant medicine under the contexts I suggest (and have experienced) has the power to warm and illuminate us when we are in the dark. Fire has the power to melt metals from ore and purify gold. But it also has the power to damage. Plant medicine works the same way.

When we realize we are working with an element that offers this much power, we must learn to approach it with humility, reverence, and prudence.

Begin with a little plant medicine. Less is more. You can always take in more medicine, but to do too much too soon can overload your senses and blast you off into other worlds, while simultaneously plunging you prematurely deep into your body and your mind.

For Sensitives and Empaths

If you are already highly sensitive and empathic and can easily feel emotions, then to add an amplifying effect via cannabis on top of those gifts can cause stimulus overload and paranoia—especially if you haven't worked with the medicine before. If this description fits you, I suggest you try small amounts of cannabis with a trusted friend or with yourself in a peaceful setting that fosters deep listening.

In his book, *Cannabis and Spirituality*, author Stephen Gray makes a powerful point, "...there's no danger of a toxic overdose with cannabis. We're talking about unwanted psychological and physiological experiences that are usually precipitated by feeling one's cocoon or ego threatened by a strong dose. Cannabis can open us up but we have to let go into that experience. You can become frightened by that opening. You may not even realize that fear is the real driving force of your distress. You may just experience physical symptoms like tightness, dizziness, exhaustion, panic attacks or nausea. Or you may fall prey to terrifying thoughts that trick you into thinking irrevocable disaster is ruining you."

What happens when we combine *Santa Maria* with yoga goes way, way beyond poses and learning fancy breathwork. This combination pierces through time, and perhaps our own preconceptions. It gives us the ability to get in contact with the ephemeral, primitive, and expansive at the same time. If you are treading these grounds for the first time, or for the first time in this way, tread gently.

Looking at Legalities

As of this writing in 2020, thirty-one states and the District of Columbia have laws legalizing marijuana in some form. But only ten states and the District of Columbia allow marijuana for recreational use. So, depending on where you are, to openly practice the use of its healing benefits through yoga or life coaching or therapy requires great discernment. We need to comply with the laws wherever we are and keep ourselves safe. Know the laws where you are partaking.

With that understood, I have read that marijuana is accepted in many different countries even if their laws don't support its use. If you plan on using marijuana as you travel, two good websites that show which states and countries are legal can be found at https://www.businessinsider.com/legal-marijuana-states-2018-1. and

https://www.thrillist.com/vice/30-places-where-weed-is-legal-cities-and-countries-with-decriminalized-marijuana.

Here in the U.S., legislation hasn't kept up with the needs of the people. But we are getting there. Where I live in

Hawaii, marijuana is only legal for medicinal purposes—you have to get a doctor's prescription to carry a card that allows you to use, grow or purchase marijuana. I work within the framework of the laws so that I am protected. I also push the envelope, as I realize how many of us desperately need this medicine.

My Sacred Plant Medicine Yoga Classes are open to everyone, whether they have a medical marijuana card or not. To keep within the law, and still offer the plant medicine yoga and life coaching, I've set it up so that those that have a card can partake on the premises in a circle as ceremony. Those that don't have a card partake privately in their car or at their home *before* class. I am not fully protected under the current laws to teach this practice. Sometimes a student doesn't have a medical marijuana card and they partake and do the yoga. If you plan on offering marijuana yoga publicly, know your laws. Talk to an attorney who can help you fully understand what you need to do to stay protected. I find this is the best way to honor your calling, while staying within the parameters of what is legal. I remain optimistic that the cannabis laws everywhere will soon reflect the growing awareness and needs of so many of us.

Overuse/Addiction

As more states continue to open marijuana laws for recreational use, critics and the legitimately concerned warn that people could become addicted to cannabis. Frankly, we sadly live in a country and a time where we potentially can become addicted to almost anything that makes us temporarily feel better. Some things are easier to become addicted to than others: food, drugs, coffee, shopping, sex, chocolate, and social media! There are bound to be people who will over-use cannabis and/or abuse it and/or become psychologically addicted to it. Addictions are how we mask pain or uncomfortable feelings. We can become addicted to anything that boosts our brain neurotransmitters.

Those of us living in the United States and Canada have become a society that can get addicted to something as basic to our survival as eating. We can become addicted to shopping, to love, to sex, to alcohol, to the internet, gaming, gambling and even our telephones. Doesn't it make sense we could possibly become addicted to marijuana? That doesn't mean it doesn't have far-reaching benefits for us and, just like eating, we need to develop healthy boundaries about how much we consume.

When we treat cannabis as sacred, we find this plant medicine can actually shed light on our addictions and can help us look at the underlying, unmet needs we are trying to fill, or the feelings we are trying to dodge or muffle. We need to practice discernment.

I have found the frequent use of marijuana as a sacrament delivers diminishing returns. Partaking too frequently in plant medicine lessens its ability to deliver the insights— and one does need more to reach the same heights. I take frequent breaks from the plant altogether.

Recently, I experimented with micro-dosing a small amount of cannabis every day for a month to see what it was like. Many people are daily users and I wanted to see what it did for me, but by day three, I woke up feeling as though I was living in a green haze. Instead of the medicine bringing clarity, I felt dulled.

My short experiment ended with me confirming that I need to do what keeps my nervous system in balance. Keep checking in with *you* as you work with the plant and see what its effects are on your nervous system. And, I highly recommend Stephen Gray's book *Cannabis and Spirituality*, for more information on ways to work with dosing and dosage.

Appendix

ACTIONS YOU CAN TAKE TO SAVE THE EARTH

"We need enlightenment, not just individually but collectively, to save the planet. We need to awaken ourselves. We need to practice mindfulness if we want to have a future, if we want to save ourselves and the planet." —Thich Nhat Hanh

I added some of my own practices and ideas to this thoughtful list of earth-saving actions, which was compiled by Katie Lambert and Sarah Gleim and was published at this link: https://science.howstuffworks.com/environmental/green-science/save-earth-top-ten1.htm:

1. Get Outside and Enjoy Her

How do you show a child you love them? You give them your attention. It is the same with Mother Earth. Look and marvel at her beauty. Play on her grass. Swim or wade in her waters. Climb her mountains. Climb her trees. Enjoy her! Let yourself feel gratitude for the gifts she continuously gives. Get Outside.

2. Conserve Water

The little things can make a big difference. Every time you turn off the water while you're brushing your teeth, you're doing something good. And stop drinking bottled water. Switch to filtered tap water. You'll save a ton of cash and help reduce a ton of plastic waste in the process.

3. Be Car-conscious

When you decide you need to buy your next car, go electric. Or, think twice and consider if you really need the purchase. If you can, stay off the road two days a week or more. You'll reduce greenhouse gas emissions by an average of 1,590 pounds (721 kilograms) per year. It's easier than you think. You can combine your errands—hit the school, grocery store and dog daycare in one trip. And talk to your boss about teleworking. It's a boon for you and your company. But being car conscious also means maintaining your car on a regular basis. You can improve your gas mileage by 0.6 percent to 3 percent by keeping your tires inflated to the proper pressure and be sure to make necessary repairs if your car fails emission.

4. Walk, Bike or Take Public Transit

Walking and biking are obvious ways to reduce greenhouse gases. Plus, you'll get some good cardio and burn some calories while you do it. If you live in an area that's not walkable, take advantage of your local mass transit if you can. Or carpool. Even one car off the road makes a difference.

5. Reduce, Reuse, Recycle

You can help reduce pollution just by putting that can in the recycling bin. It really does make a difference. Paper, too. Case in point: If an office building of 7,000 workers recycled all of its office paper waste for a year, it would be the equivalent of taking almost 400 cars off the road. But you can also take reusable bags to the grocery, and avoid using disposable plates, spoons, glass, cups, and napkins. They create huge amounts of waste. And buy products that are made of recycled materials. It all makes a difference.

6. Give Composting a Try

In 2015 (the last year figures were available), Americans generated 262.4 million tons (238 metric tons) of trash. Only 23.4 million tons (21.2 metric tons) of that was composted. Some was recycled and some was combusted for energy, but almost half of it — 137.7 million tons (124.9 metric tons) — ended up in the landfill. Imagine if you could divert more of that to your own compost? It would help reduce the amount of solid waste you produce, and what eventually winds up in your local landfill. Plus, compost makes a great natural fertilizer.

7. Switch to LEDs

Compact fluorescent light bulbs (CFLs) are great. They can last 10 times longer than incandescent bulbs and they use at least two-thirds less energy, but even CFLS have issues. They're hard to dispose of because they contain mercury. Enter light-emitting diode, or LED bulbs. They emit light in a very narrow band wavelength so they're super energy-efficient. Start replacing your old incandescent bulbs with LED bulbs now (if you haven't already). They do cost more than CFLs and incandescents, but equivalent LED bulbs can last around 25,000 hours compared to the 1,000 hours that incandescent bulb might have lasted.

8. Live Energy Wise

Make your home more energy efficient (and save money). Your home's windows are responsible for 25 to 30 percent of residential heat gain and heat loss. If they're old and inefficient, consider replacing them. Also, be sure your home has proper insulation. Insulation is measured in terms of its thermal resistance or R-value—the higher the R-value, the more effective the insulation. The amount of insulation your home needs depends on the climate, type of HVAC system, and where you're adding the insulation. Smaller things you can do right away include replacing your air filter regularly so your HVAC system doesn't have to work overtime. Keep your window treatments closed when it's extremely hot or cold outside. You can also consider installing a programmable thermostat like <u>Nest</u> so your system isn't running (and wasting energy) when you're not home.

9. Eat Sustainable Foods

Today, large-scale food production accounts for as much as <u>25 percent of the greenhouse emissions</u>. So how do you eat sustainably? Choosing food from farmers that aim to conserve the natural resources and have as little impact on the land as possible. But even buying as much as you can from local farmers makes a difference. Eating more whole grains, vegetables, fruits and nuts, and less red meats and processed foods makes a difference as well. Grow your own fruits and vegetables. You can grow a garden!

10. Plant a Tree (or Two)

In 2018, the United Nations' Intergovernmental Panel on Climate Change (IPCC) report, the U.N. suggests an additional 2.5 billion acres (1 billion hectares) of forest in the world could limit global warming to 2.7 degrees Fahrenheit (1.5 degrees Celsius) by 2050. That's a lot of trees, but you could plant one or two, right? One young tree can absorb CO_2 at a rate of 13 pounds (5 kilograms) per tree. Every. Single. Year. And that's just an itty-bitty baby tree. Once that tree reaches about 10 years old, it's at its most productive stage of carbon storage. Then it can absorb 48 pounds (21 kilograms) of CO2 per year. Trees also remove all other kinds of junk from the air, including sulfur dioxide, nitrogen oxides and small particles. So, go ahead, plant a tree. It's good for everybody.

11. Give Up Plastics

The statistics are shocking: People around the world buy 1 million plastic drinking bottles *every minute*, and use up to *5 trillion* single-use plastic bags every year. Humans are addicted to plastic, and hardly any of it — about 9 percent— gets recycled. A staggering 8 million tons (7.25 metric tons) ends up in the ocean every year. Break the cycle. Stop buying bottled water. Say no to plastic shopping bags and use cloth bags instead. Don't use plastic straws. Drink from a reusable cup instead of a plastic one. Avoiding plastic can divert a ton of waste from the oceans and landfill.

12. Practice Gratitude

Lastly and most importantly, I have found that being grateful for everything in my life allows everything that's beautiful in it to grow and flourish. When I am grateful, I express love for all that I have, see and know. Taking the time to enjoy and play and have fun on the earth is one of the biggest ways I show my love for her. I feel so, so lucky to be able to go the ocean and jump in the waves and hike up a volcano and dive behind a waterfall. When we are aware of what we have, we take better care of it! Love what you have and let the rest go.

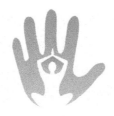

BRENT'S RECIPE FOR HOLY ANOINTING OIL

Exodus 30: 23-25 -1446 BCE

Then the Lord said to Moses, "Take the following fine spices: 500 shekels of liquid myrrh, half as much (that is, 250 shekels) of fragrant cinnamon, 250 shekels of fragrant calamus [cannabis], 500 shekels of cassia–all according to the sanctuary shekel–and a hint of olive oil. Make these into a sacred anointing oil, a fragrant blend, the work of a perfumer. It will be the sacred anointing oil."

Thanks to science, we can now isolate properties within this sacred timeless biblical recipe of herbs and oil and break down what each does and ascertain its exact healing potential. Some of these herbs are antiviral, some anti-fungal, while another is antibacterial. Combined, these herbs make a powerful elixir of healing medicinal properties that have

181

been handed down for thousands of years. This is a forceful, potent, and sacred healing oil from Nature.

What You Will Need

A food scale

Coffee grinder

12 inch diameter pot (10–12 quart) no lid

Fine mesh strainer

8-inch glass bowl that holds at least 7 cups

10-inch diameter glass bowl

Your favorite mindful high vibrational intentional music

Ingredients

2.5 gm top shelf flower (herb)

2 cups coconut oil (do not use MCT oil) this works better with an oil that can solidify when it is chilled. (see below for how to infuse)

7 cups water

1/2 teaspoon cinnamon essential oil

1/2 teaspoon frankincense essential oil

1/2 teaspoon myrrh essential oil

1/2 teaspoon rosemary essential oil

1/2 teaspoon orange essential oil

Cinnamon is loaded with powerful antioxidants, such as polyphenols. It is excellent to use to cleanse the air, help kill molds and boost the immune system. It is antimicrobial and is great for heart health and helps to combat oxidative stress with its antioxidant capabilities.

Frankincense helps boost immune system function and prevent illness.

This includes controlling bleeding, speeding up the wound-healing process, improving oral health, fighting inflammatory conditions such as <u>arthritis</u>, and improving uterine health. Studies have suggested that certain substances in frankincense may be useful as a cancer treatment and that frankincense benefits extend to immune-enhancing abilities that may help destroy dangerous bacteria, viruses, and even cancers.

Myrrh is a great analgesic, anti-inflammatory, antiviral, anti-fungal, antiseptic, anti-parasitic, anti-catarrhal and it is known for its anti-infectious properties as well. It can help uplift the mind, nourish and rejuvenate the skin and it has potent antioxidant abilities. Myrrh oil is excellent for use to improve gum health and of course, was a gift presented to baby Jesus from the Magi. This powerful essential oil can also help support good sleep patterns, help with wound soothing, and has been found to be inhibitory on five tumor cell lines helping to induce apoptosis.

Rosemary Though most of this research is preliminary, studies note that this essential oil may boost your health by improving mental focus and memory, fighting hair loss, relieving pain and inflammation, repelling certain insects and easing stress.

Orange essential oil contains all-natural antimicrobial properties and helps eliminate toxins from the body. It stimulates lymphatic action to promote balance in water processes and detoxification. It is a natural remedy for high blood pressure and has anti-inflammatory properties. Orange oil reduces anxiety, boosts mood and is a natural anti-depressant.

Cannabis offers relief of chronic pain and improves lung capacity. It can aid in weight loss and regulate and prevent diabetes, fight cancer and help treat depression. Cannabis shows promise in autism treatment, regulating seizures, mending bones and helping with ADHD and ADD, as well as treatment for glaucoma and alleviating anxiety. It may slow the development of Alzheimer's disease and helps with PTSD symptoms. People with Crohn's disease or ulcerative colitis can find some relief with the use of cannabis.

For those that have Parkinson's disease, cannabis can help reduce tremors and pain while also helping promote sleep. It has also shown to improve motor skills in patients and helps with alcoholism.

Let's Get Started

1. Turn on your favorite high vibration music.

2. Put water into a pot and set to slight simmer/boil (just barely boiling) add coconut oil to water. Add ground flower to simmering water/oil Simmer uncovered for one hour, stirring every 5 minutes.

3. Pour contents of pot through strainer into 6-inch glass bowl.

4. Use backside of a spoon to press oil out of flower that's in strainer. Use rubber spoon to clean out the pot through strainer.

5. The THC is in the oil. (You can save the leftover mash for spaghetti sauce or baked goods, etc.).

6. Cover bowl and refrigerate for 6 hours or until the oil has solidified into a hockey puck shape.

7. Put hockey puck into 10-inch bowl, let it melt (microwave for 20 seconds), this will be the base for your anointing oil.

8. Add 1/2 teaspoon of myrrh, 1/2 teaspoon of frankincense, 1/2 teaspoon of rosemary, 1/2 teaspoon of cinnamon, and 1/2 teaspoon of orange essential oils.

9. Mix well.

Pour into smaller bottles as desired. Offer the aroma first. Most people love the scent, but if they don't appreciate it, don't anoint them. Why? Because once it's ON a person— it's *IN* the person.

Offer a prayer or a blessing to set a high and healing intention. Then apply a small amount, an "underdose." Put a few drops on the inner wrist, pulse-points. Then rub wrists together. Then put about ten drops on the crown of the head, as in "anoint your head with oil." Namaste.

Recipe for Bhang Lassi

Ingredients

1/2 oz. Cannabis

2 Cups warm coconut, hemp or almond milk

3/8 Cups maple syrup or other sugar substitute

1 tbsp or more of canned Coconut cream

1 tbsp Almonds, chopped

1/8 tsp Powdered ginger

1 pinch Garam masala

1/2 tsp Grenadine

1 cup Water

How To Make It

1. Bring water to a boil in a teapot, and add the cannabis to it.

2. Brew for about 7 to 10 minutes, then strain into a bowl.

3. Gradually grind the strained cannabis along with 2 tbsp of milk using a mortar and pestle; repeat this process several times.

4. Strain the milk into another bowl and keep aside.

5. Add a little more milk to the cannabis and grind it along with the almonds, repeat this several times.

6. Strain the liquid through your sieve to remove the excess cannabis plant matter, and pour the milk, coconut cream, grenadine, and water into one pan.

7. Add ginger, maple syrup, and garam masala, bringing to a boil while stirring continuously.

8. Take the mixture off the heat. Once it is at a reasonable temperature, place it in the fridge to continue cooling for a few hours.

9. Your bhang lassi is ready to serve! Bom Shiva!

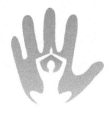

ABOUT THE AUTHOR

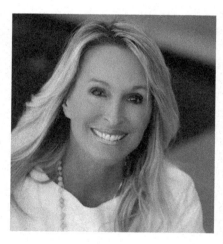

BRE WOLFE is an inspirational speaker, a compassionate spiritual teacher, Certified Integrated Life Coach, an internationally acclaimed YOGA NIDRA AMRIT instructor, Reiki Practitioner, and author. She has been featured on numerous local and national television shows as a news anchor and notable personality. Her deep spiritual journey lead her to discover a body of inner work that illuminated her spirit and soul so she could assist others to live radiant lives.

Bre believes that each of us can (and should) reconnect to our soul to unlock our full potential and explore infinite possibilities. She helps others create a luminous vision for their life with concrete actions to wake up vast internal gifts. This higher frequency work gracefully shifts one and reconnects them to soul-body alignment, allowing them to remember WHO they are and HOW they want to shine their lights!

Bre lives her passion as *her life has become her message.* She created 'Sacred Plant Medicine Yoga and Journeys', as conduits of light for planet Earth's healing and protection. "We uplift and heal everything around us as channelers of higher vibrations and frequencies. We protect all species on the planet and live and play in harmony using ancient wisdom teachings and tools to clear anything that blocks the flow of higher light frequencies. We playfully help others achieve freedom, adventure, joyful, illuminated personal transformation and connection to their true essence."

Bre has created an interactive website for your enjoyment and participation with other readers of *BREATHE*. This interactive website offers support, fun, community, and great mystical wisdom. Please go to BreWolfe.com/Breathgiving (https://www.brewolfe.com/Breathgiving) to download other gifts that will support your journey to wholeness in addition to this book's content.

Bre Wolfe lives in Maui, Hawaii with her husband, Brent, and dog Yogi. They have a beautiful, blended family with six adult children who are a constant source of inspiration. She lives her message and can help you magically turn your life around so you are living your life's purpose.

Made in USA - North Chelmsford, MA
1201410_9780998320946
11.30.2020 1618